ECGs for the Emergency Physician 1

ECGs for the Emergency Physician 2

Amal Mattu, University of Maryland Medical Center, Maryland, USA
William Brady, University of Virginia Medical Center, Charlottesville, USA

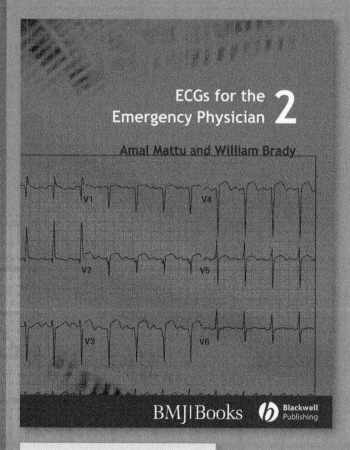

- A new companion volume to ECGs for the Emergency Physician 1, with a completely new set of examples aimed at qualified physicians needing to advance their skills

- A unique format, presenting random examples of ECGs for interpretation

- Split into two levels of difficulty: intermediate and advanced

- Focuses on emergency situations, with more emphasis on dysrhythmias in this volume

ISBN 9781405157018 • Paperback
232 pages • February 2008

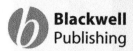
Blackwell
Publishing

To order or view a sample chapter visit
www.blackwellpublishing.com/9781405157018

ECGs for the Emergency Physician 1

Amal Mattu

Director, Emergency Medicine Residency Program, Co-Director, Emergency Medicine/Internal Medicine Combined Residency Program, University of Maryland School of Medicine, Baltimore, Maryland, USA

William Brady

Associate Professor, Vice Chair, and Program Director, Department of Emergency Medicine University of Virginia Health System, Charlottesville, Virginia, USA
and
Medical Director, Charlottesville-Albermarle Rescue Squad, Charlottesville, Virginia, USA

© BMJ Publishing Group 2003
BMJ Books is an imprint of the BMJ Publishing Group

First published in 2003
22   2019
by BMJ Books, BMA House, Tavistock Square,
London WC1H 9JR

www.bmjbooks.com

British Library Cataloguing in Publication Data

A catalogue record for this book is available from the British Library

ISBN 978-0-7279-1654-9

Typeset by SIVA Math Setters, Chennai, India
Printed and bound by CPI Group (UK) Ltd, Croydon, CR0 4YY

Contents

Foreword

There has been a great need for a user friendly ECG text that fills the void between an introductory text designed for students and an advanced reference source for cardiologists. "*ECGs for the Emergency Physician*" fills this void. It is an ECG teaching and reference textbook for acute and emergency care physicians written by two specialists practicing and teaching acute and emergency care.

Drs Mattu and Brady have created an ECG text that facilitates self instruction in learning the basics, as well as the complexities, of ECG interpretation. They know that ECG interpretation requires knowledge, insight and practice. They know "the eye does not see, what the mind does not know." In order to accomplish this goal of teaching ECG interpretation, they have divided their book into two parts. In Part I, as the authors state, are the "bread and butter" ECGs of acute care. These are the ECG findings that form the core knowledge necessary for accurate ECG interpretation. In Part II they teach recognition of more subtle ECG abnormalities, which when mastered, allow the practitioner to become an expert.

The beauty of this text lies in the combining of a collection of emergency department ECGs with the authors' insights and expert observations. This book has great utility as a reference text, a bound ECG teaching file, a board review aide or a resident in emergency medicine's best friend for learning the art of advanced ECG interpretation. Its greatest value however, is for all of us who want to be both challenged and taught by 200 great electrocardiograms and their interpretations.

May the forces be with you.

Corey M Slovis
Professor of Emergency Medicine and Medicine
Chairman, Department of Emergency Medicine
Vanderbilt Medical Center
Nashville, Tennessee
Medical Director Metro Nashville Fire EMS

Preface

Emergency and other acute care physicians must be experts in the use and interpretation of the 12-lead electrocardiogram (ECG). We have prepared this text with this basic though highly important thought in mind. This text represents our effort to further the art and science of electrocardiography as practiced by emergency physicians and other acute care clinicians.

A significant number of the patients managed in the emergency department and other acute care settings present with chest pain, cardiovascular instability, or complaints related to the cardiovascular system. The known benefits of early, accurate diagnosis and rapid, appropriate treatment of cardiovascular emergencies have only reinforced the importance of physician competence in electrocardiographic interpretation. The physician is charged with the responsibility of rapid, accurate diagnosis followed by appropriate therapy delivered expeditiously. This evaluation not infrequently involves the performance of the 12-lead ECG. For example, the patient with chest pain presenting with ST-segment elevation, acute myocardial infarction must be rapidly and accurately evaluated so that appropriate therapy is offered in prompt fashion. Alternatively, the hemodynamically unstable patient with atrioventricular block similarly must be cared for in a rapid manner. In these instances as well as numerous other scenarios, resuscitative and other therapies are largely guided by information obtained from the ECG.

The electrocardiogram is used frequently in the emergency department (ED) and other acute care settings; numerous presentations may require a 12-lead electrocardiogram. For instance, the most frequent indication for ECG performance in the ED is the presence of chest pain; other complaints include dyspnea and syncope. Additional reasons for obtaining an ECG in the ED include both diagnosis-based (acute coronary syndrome, suspected pulmonary embolism, and the "dysrhythmic" patient) and system-related indications (for the "rule-out myocardial infarction" protocol, for admission purposes, and for operative clearance).[1] Regardless of the cause, the physician must be an expert in the interpretation of the 12-lead ECG. Interpretation of the ECG is as much an art as it is a science. Accurate ECG interpretation requires a sound knowledge of the electrocardiogram, both the objective criteria necessary for various diagnoses of those patients encountered in the ED as well as a thorough grasp of the various electrocardiographic waveforms and their meaning in the individual patient.

We have prepared this text for the physician who manages patients not only in the ED but also in other acute care settings – whether it be in the office, the hospital ward, critical care unit, the out-of-hospital arena, or other patient-care locale. We have used actual ECGs from patients treated in our EDs; a brief but accurate history has also been provided in each instance. In certain cases, the history may provide a clue to the diagnosis yet in other situations the clinical information will have no relationship to the final diagnosis – as is the case in the ED. We have made an effort to choose the most appropriate ECG from each patient, but as occurs in "real ED," some of the ECGs are imperfect: the evaluation is hindered by artifact, incomplete electrocardiographic sampling, etc. We have also provided the ECGs in a random fashion, much the way actual patients present to the emergency department. We have endeavored to reproduce the reality of the ED when the reader uses this text to expand their knowledge of the 12-lead electrocardiogram and how it relates to patient care.

The reader is advised to read the clinical history provided for each ECG and then, much as the clinician would interpret the electrocardiogram in the ED, review the 12-lead ECG. After a clinically focused review of the ECG, the reader is then able to review the interpretation. This ECG text has been constructed in two basic sections. The first half of the text contains ECGs that we feel represent the "bread and butter" of emergency electrocardiography – the core material with which we feel that the acute care physician must be thoroughly familiar. These ECGs were chosen because they represent common electrocardiographic diagnoses that all emergency physicians should know. This section is prepared primarily for the physician-in-training (for example, the emergency medicine resident) though practicing physicians will also benefit from reviewing the material. The second half of the text is composed of ECGs that are more challenging. The electrocardiographic diagnoses are more difficult to establish and will often be on subtle findings. In some cases, the ECGs in this section were chosen not necessarily because of the related level of difficulty but because of subtle teaching points found, which are likely to be beyond the level of the physician-in-training.

It is also crucial to understand that this text is not intended for the "beginner in ECG interpretation". The text, **in essence an electrocardiographic teaching file**, is intended for the physician who possesses a sound, basic understanding of electrocardiography yet desires additional practice and review – a review which is highly clinically pertinent. The electrocardiography beginner is advised to begin by reading through one of the many outstanding books that have previously been written for novice students prior to studying this teaching file.

One last point must also be stressed to the reader of this text. Diagnostic criteria for various electrocardiographic diagnoses vary somewhat amongst authors. Therefore, in an effort to standardize the interpretations used in this text, we chose to use the following two references as the "gold standard" for electrocardiographic interpretations: Chou and Knilans' *Electrocardiography in Clinical Practice: Adult and Pediatric* and Galen's *Marriott's Practical Electrocardiography*.[2,3]

References
1. Brady W, Adams M, Perron A, Martin M. The impact of the 12-lead electrocardiogram in the evaluation of the emergency department patient. *Ann Emerg Med* (accepted for publication/publication pending).
2. Chou T-C, Knilans TK. *Electrocardiography in Clinical Practice: Adult and Pediatric 4th edn*. Philadelphia, PA: WB Saunders Company, 1996.
3. Galen SW. *Marriott's Practical Electrocardiography 10th edn*. Philadelphia, PA: Lippincott Williams & Wilkins, 2001.

Dedications

This work is dedicated to my wife, Sejal, for her tremendous patience and never-ending support; to my son, Nikhil, for constantly reminding me of the priorities in life; to the Emergency Department staff at Mercy Medical Center in Baltimore for their friendship and their ECG contributions; to the faculty and residents of the University of Maryland Emergency Medicine Residency Program for providing the main inspiration for this work; to Mary Banks and BMJ Books for supporting and believing in this work; to Dr Bill Brady for his mentorship, friendship, and commitment to teaching and education; and to emergency physicians around the world – may your dedication to learning continue to strengthen our specialty and improve patient care.

Amal Mattu
Director, Emergency Medicine Residency Program
Co-Director, Emergency Medicine/Internal Medicine Combined Residency Program
University of Maryland School of Medicine
Baltimore, Maryland
USA

I would like to thank my wife, King, for her love, support, wise counsel, and patience – none of this effort would be possible without her; my children, Lauren, Anne, Chip, and Katherine, for being wonderful and my primary inspiration; my parents, Bill and Joann Brady, for all that they have done and continue to do; the Emergency Medicine Residents (past, present, and future) at the University of Virginia, for their hard work, astronomical dedication, and inspiration – all directed at our patients and the specialty of Emergency Medicine; Dr Marcus Martin, Chair of Emergency Medicine at the University of Virginia, for his support, guidance, and mentorship; and my co-author, Dr Amal Mattu, for his dedicated effort on this book in particular and his dedication to Emergency Medicine education in general – a true gentleman, talented clinician, and distinguished scholar.

William Brady
Associate Professor, Vice Chair, and Program Director
Department of Emergency Medicine
University of Virginia Health System
Charlottesville, Virginia
USA
and
Medical Director, Charlottesville-Albermarle
Rescue Squad, Charlottesville, Virginia,
USA

Part 1

Case histories

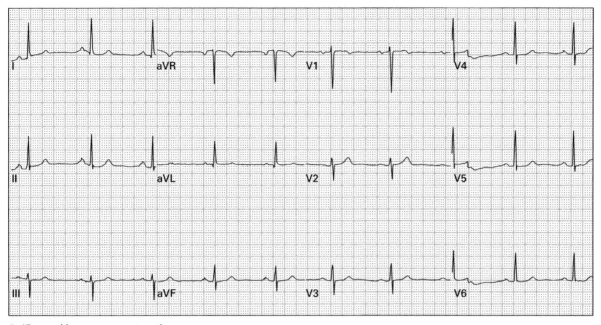

1. 45 year old woman, asymptomatic

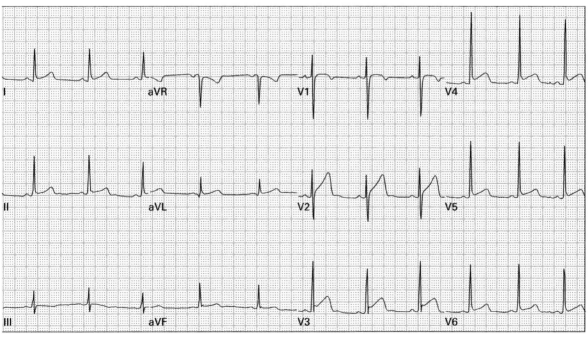

2. 24 year old man with chest ache after lifting weights

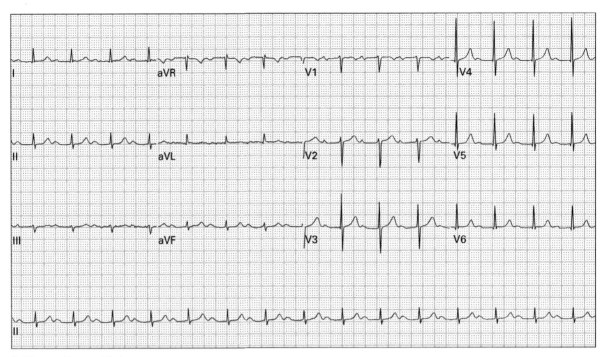

3. 76 year old man with dyspnea

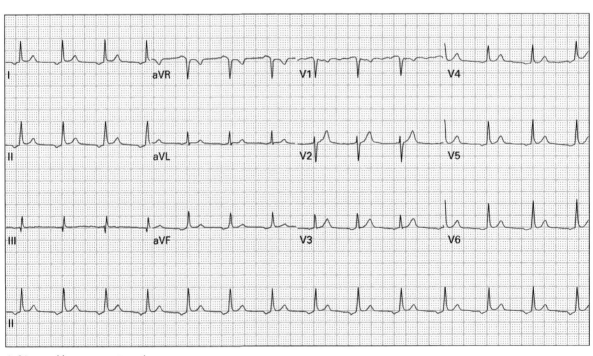

4. 64 year old man, asymptomatic

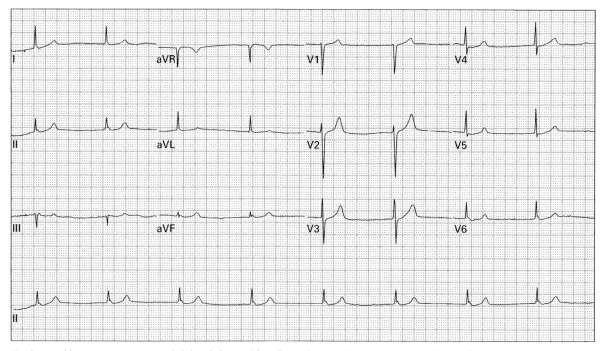

5. 48 year old woman reports severe lightheadedness with walking; she recently started a new medication for hypertension

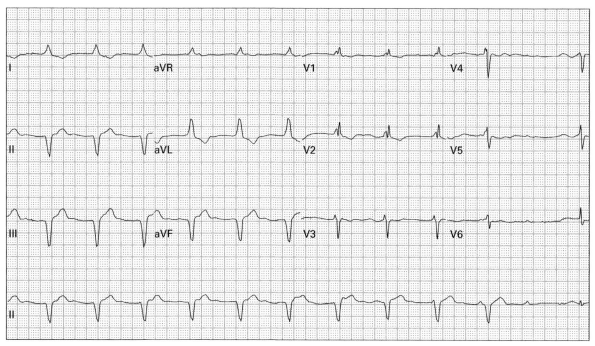

6. 79 year old man 45 minutes after receiving thrombolytic therapy for acute myocardial infarction; currently pain-free

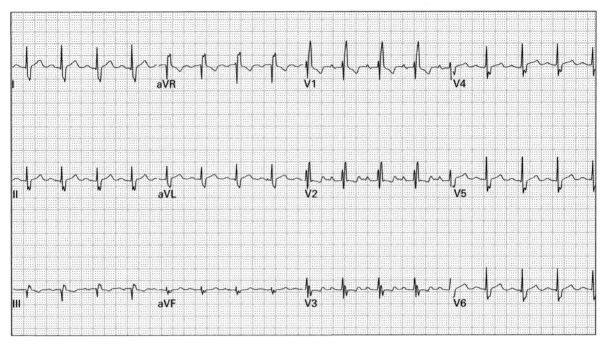

7. 43 year old man, asymptomatic

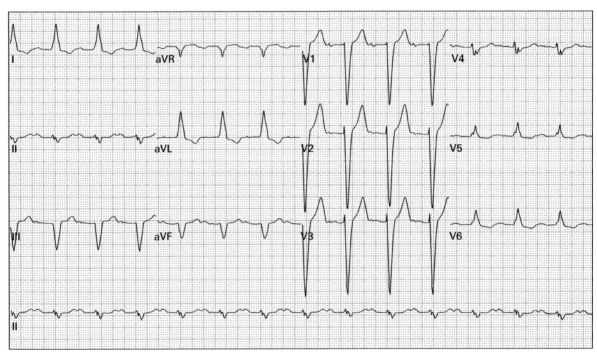

8. 82 year old man recently increased his dose of a beta-receptor blocking medication; he now reports exertional lightheadedness

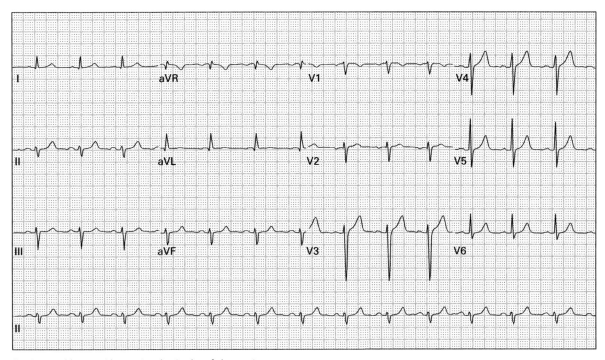

9. 49 year old man with occasional episodes of chest pain

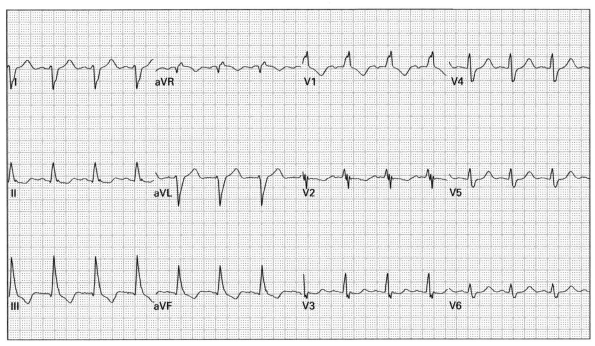

10. 65 year old woman with a long history of smoking presents for treatment of an emphysema exacerbation

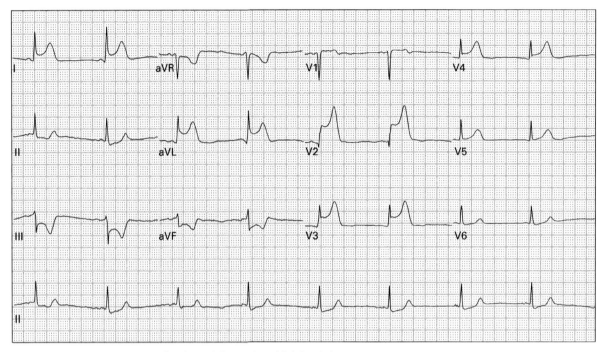

11. 54 year old woman complains of midsternal chest pain and lightheadedness

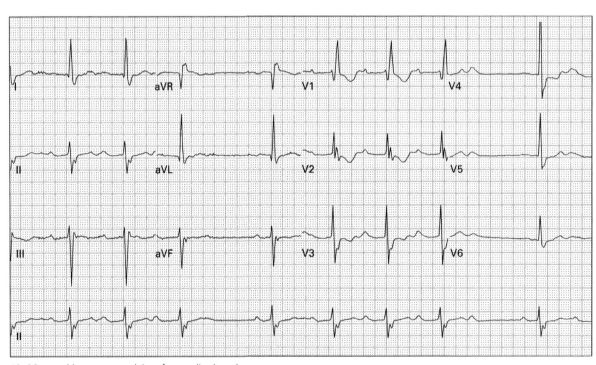

12. 86 year old woman complains of generalized weakness

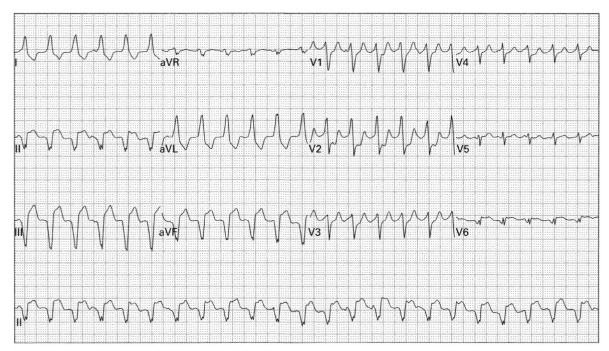

13. 61 year old man with palpitations and lightheadedness

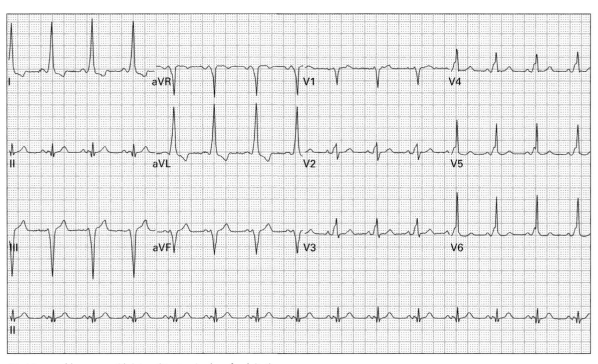

14. 44 year old woman with intermittent episodes of palpitations

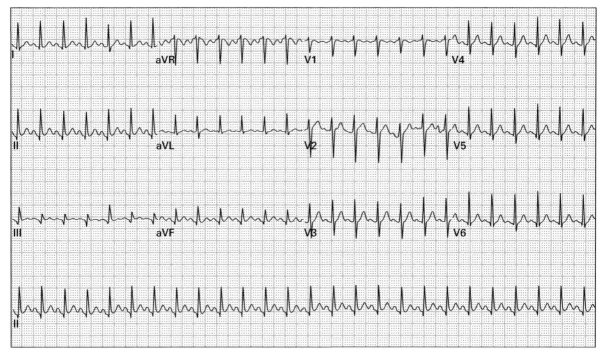

15. 24 year old pregnant woman with three days of frequent vomiting

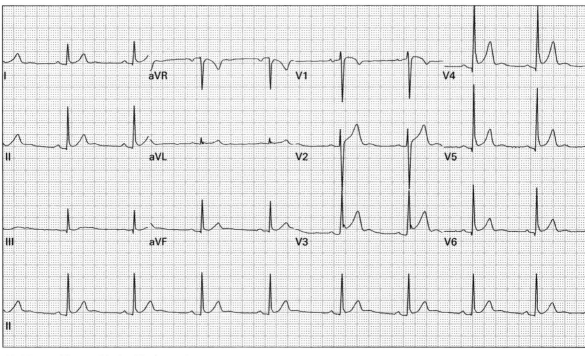

16. 37 year old man with pleuritic chest pain

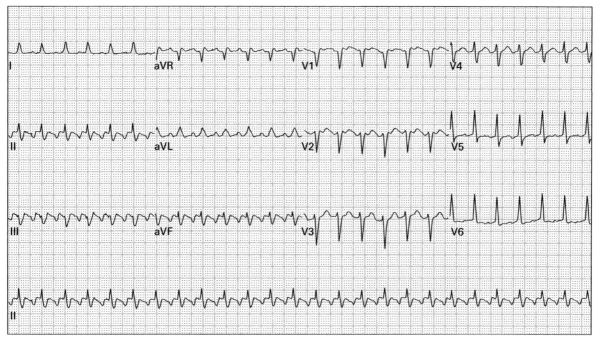

17. 63 year old man with palpitations and lightheadedness

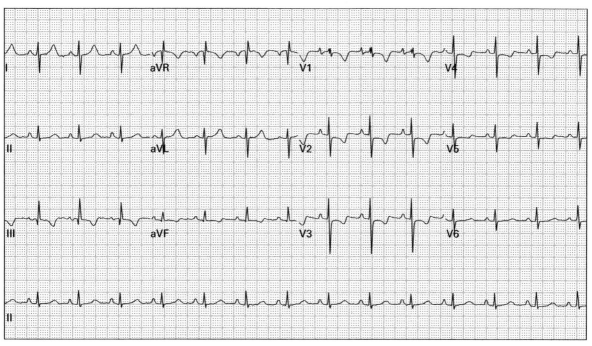

18. 33 year old obese man with sharp chest pain and dyspnea

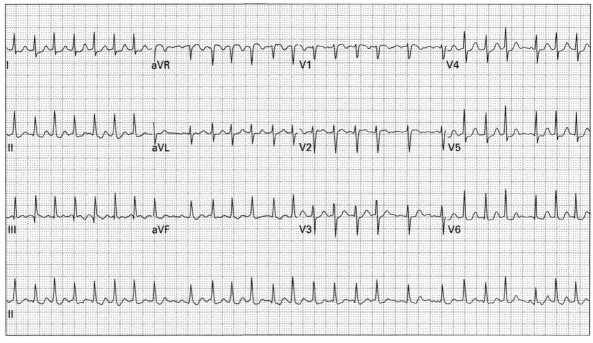

19. 81 year old woman with palpitations and generalized weakness

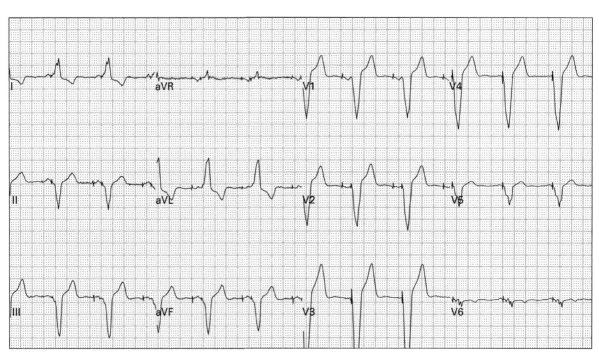

20. 61 year old man, asymptomatic

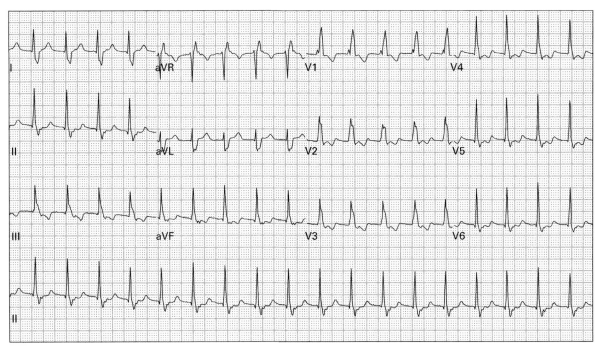

21. 57 year old woman with mild chest pain and palpitations

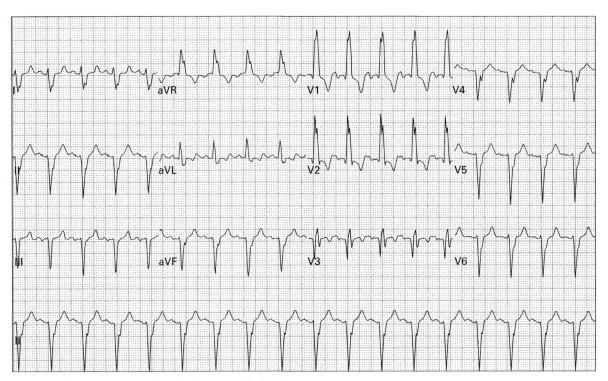

22. 75 year old man presents with cough, dyspnea, and wheezing

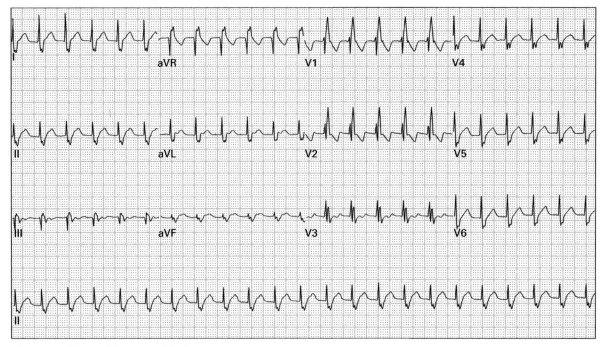

23. 43 year old man with severe palpitations

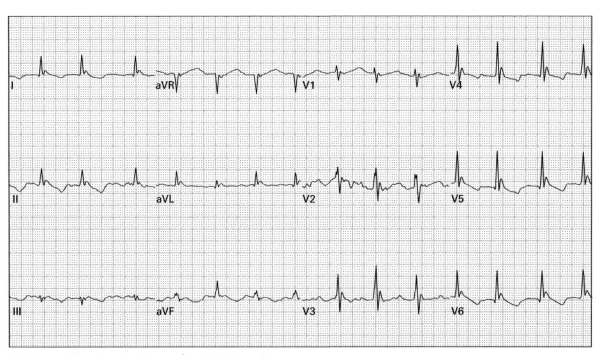

24. 52 year old homeless, alcoholic man found lying in an alley

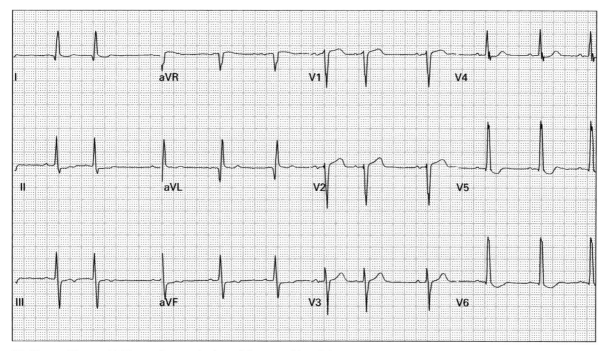

25. 68 year old man with history of congestive heart failure complains of dyspnea

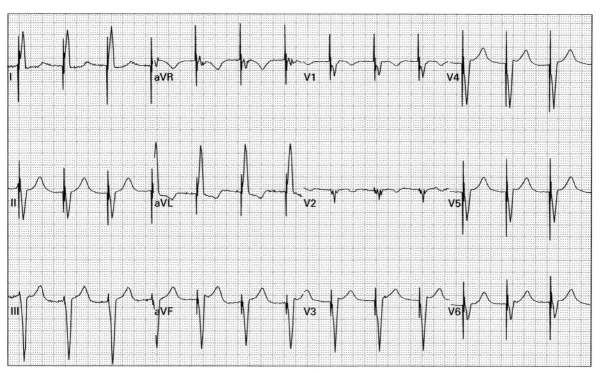

26. 85 year old woman reports a recent syncopal episode

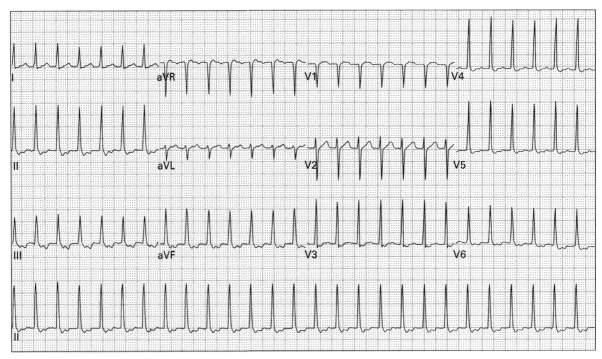

27. 40 year old woman with palpitations and lightheadedness

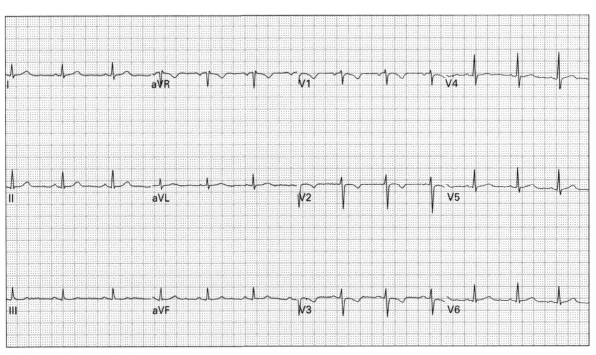

28. 35 year old woman with dyspnea

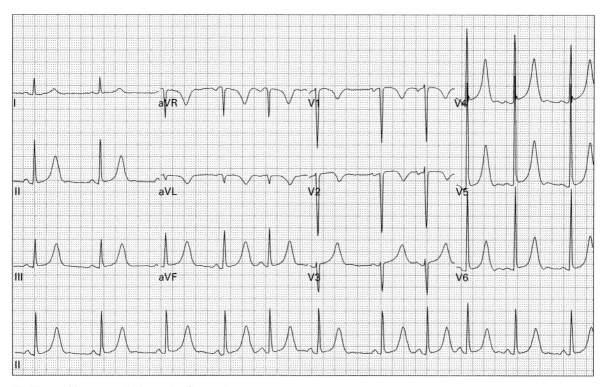

29. 41 year old woman with chest pain after cocaine use

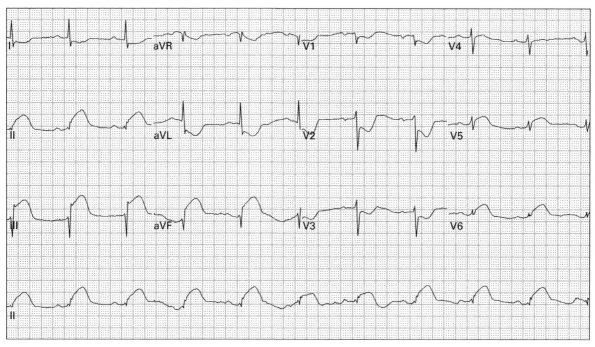

30. 57 year old man with chest pressure and diaphoresis

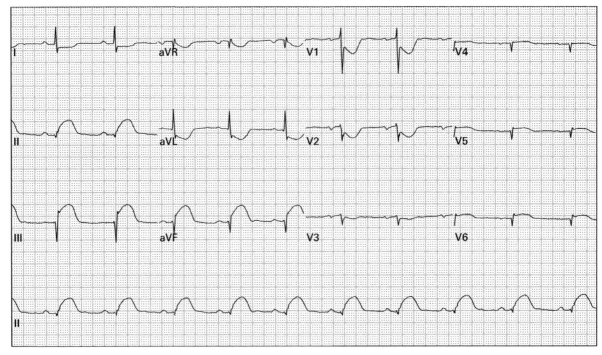

31. 57 year old man with chest pressure and diaphoresis (right-sided precordial leads)

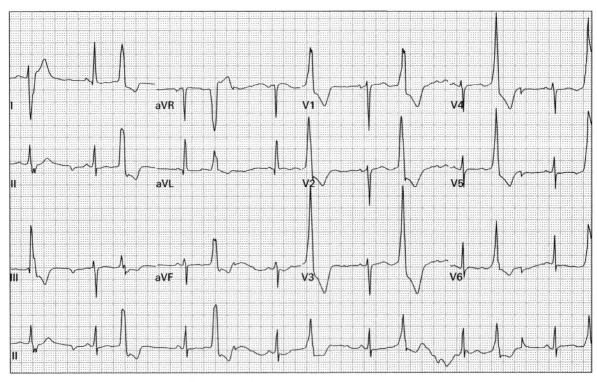

32. 60 year old woman with acute onset of expressive aphasia

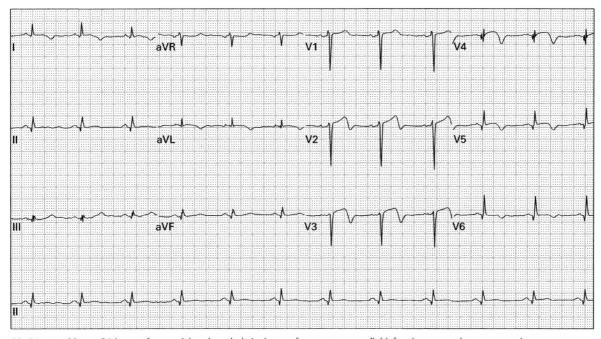

33. 54 year old man 24 hours after receiving thrombolytic therapy for acute myocardial infarction; currently asymptomatic

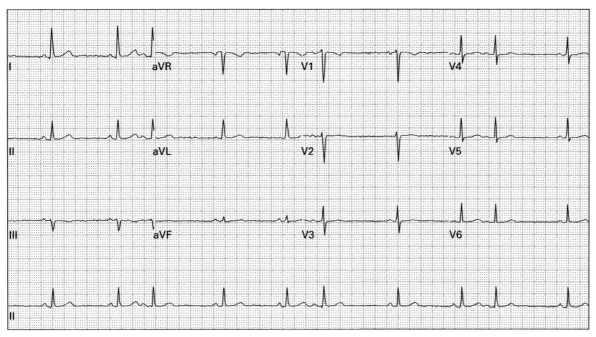

34. 41 year old woman with nausea and vomiting

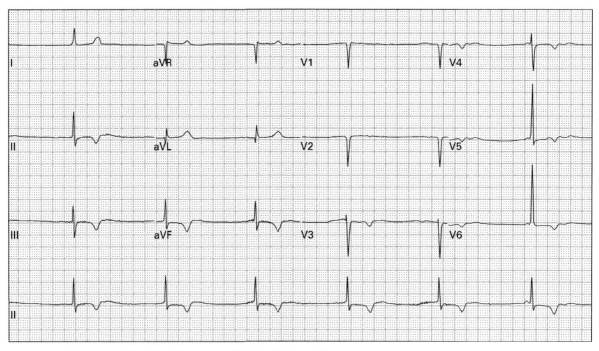

35. 75 year old woman accidentally took too many of her beta-blocker tablets

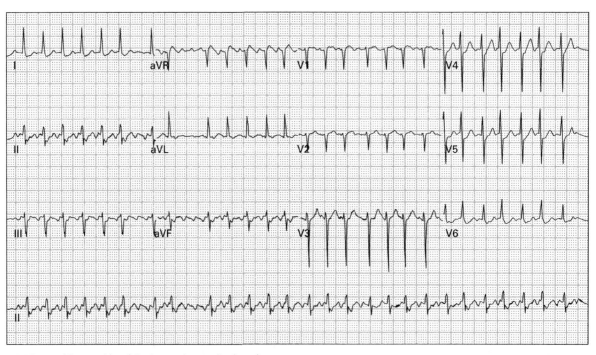

36. 68 year old man with palpitations and generalized weakness

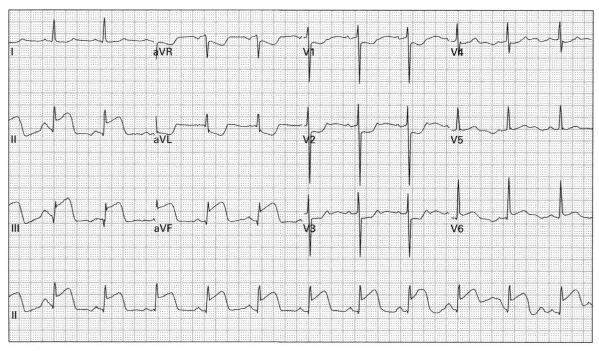

37. 38 year old man with chest pain, nausea, and diaphoresis

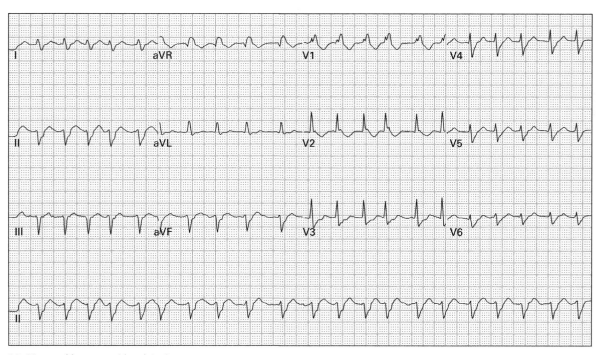

38. 62 year old woman with palpitations

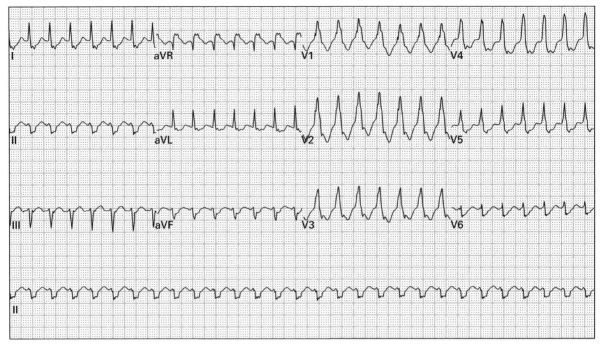

39. 74 year old man with chest pain and palpitations

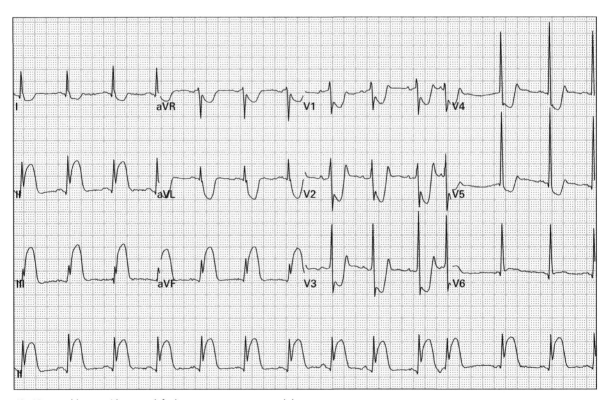

40. 45 year old man with severe left chest pressure, nausea, and dyspnea

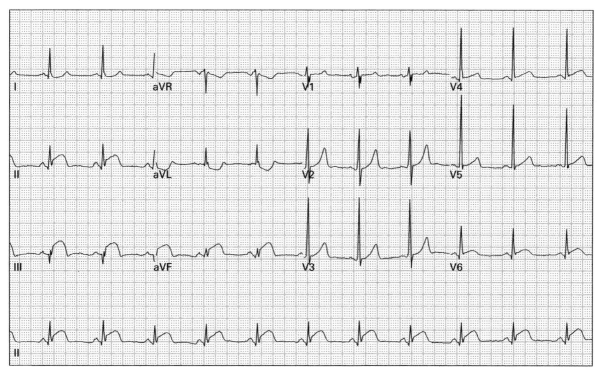

41. 45 year old man with left chest pressure

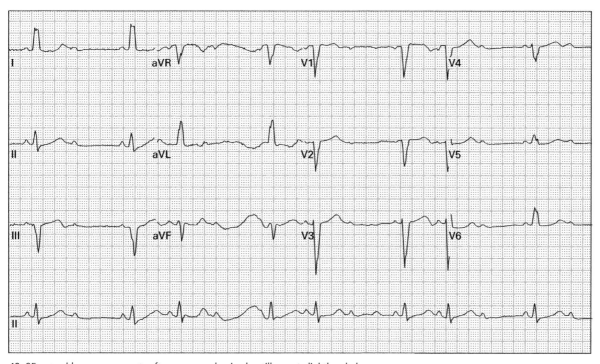

42. 85 year old woman presents after a syncopal episode, still reports lightheadedness

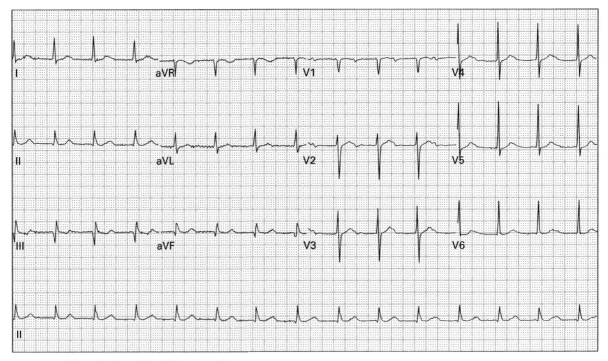

43. 81 year old man being admitted for pneumonia

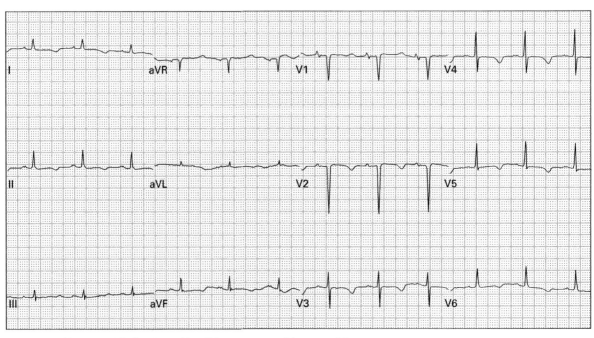

44. 71 year old woman with chronic renal insufficiency presents with carpopedal spasm

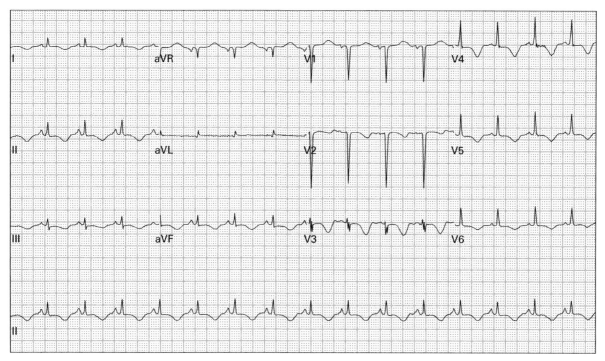

45. 46 year old man with chest and left arm pain, vomiting, and diaphoresis

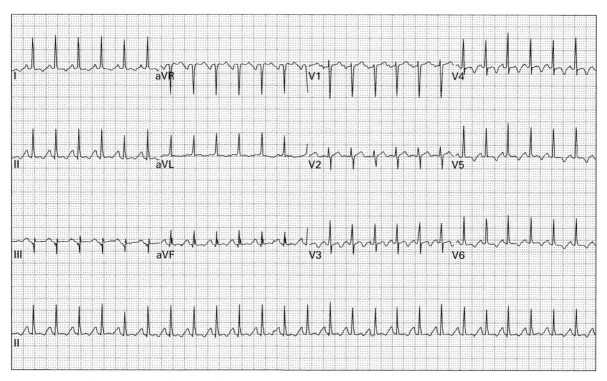

46. 53 year old diabetic woman with four days of nausea, vomiting, and lightheadedness

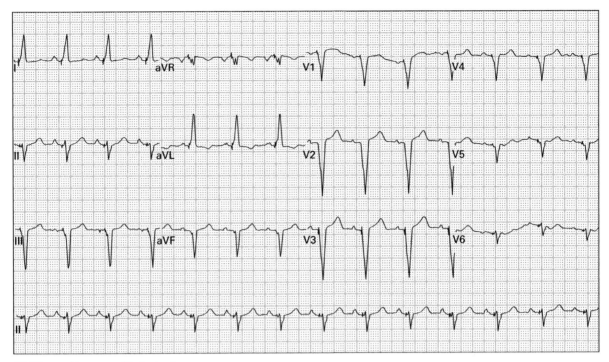

47. 85 year old woman with chest pain

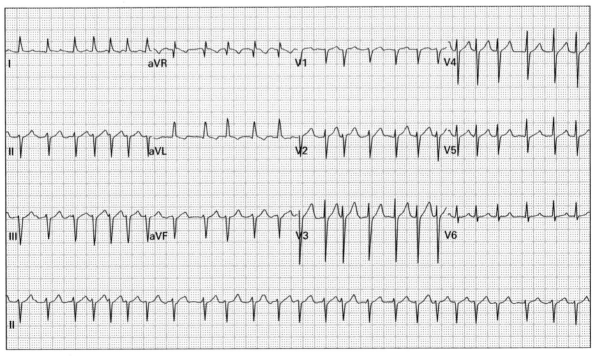

48. 66 year old man with severe lightheadedness and diaphoresis

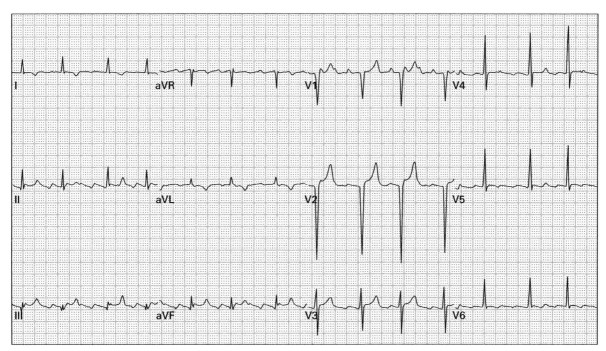

49. 58 year old man with congestive heart failure reports increasing dyspnea and lower extremity edema

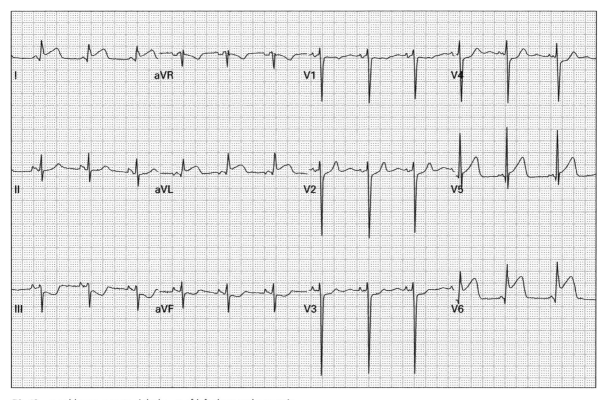

50. 43 year old man reports eight hours of left chest and arm pain

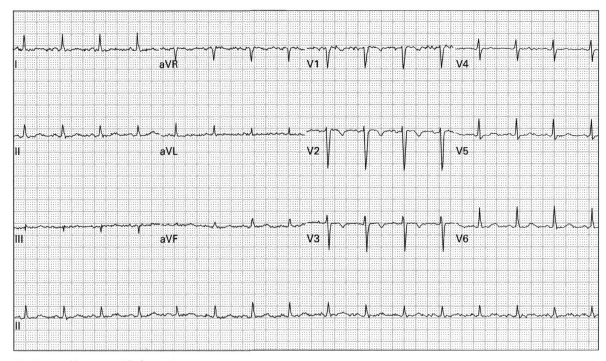

51. 52 year old woman with chest pain

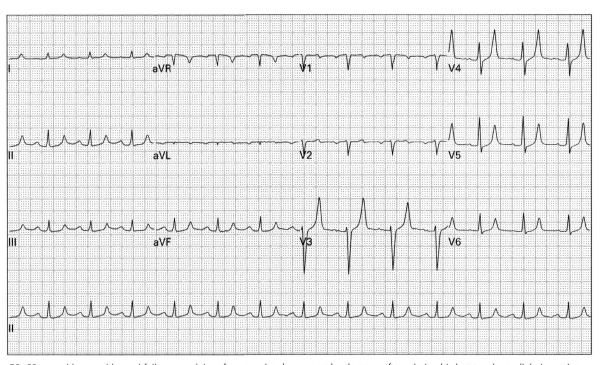

52. 62 year old man with renal failure complains of progressive dyspnea and orthopnea after missing his last two hemodialysis sessions

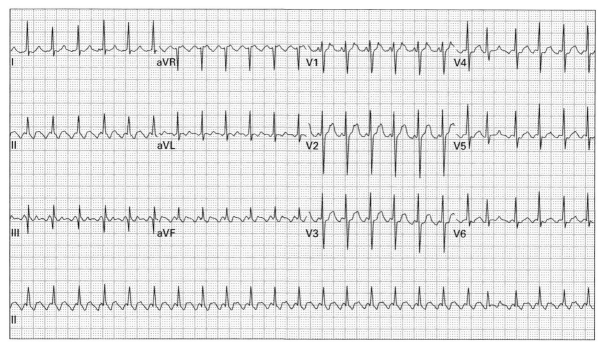

53. 47 year old man with palpitations and dyspnea

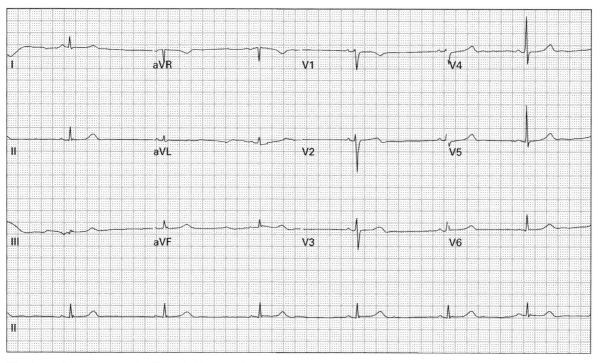

54. 48 year old woman presents after a clonidine overdose

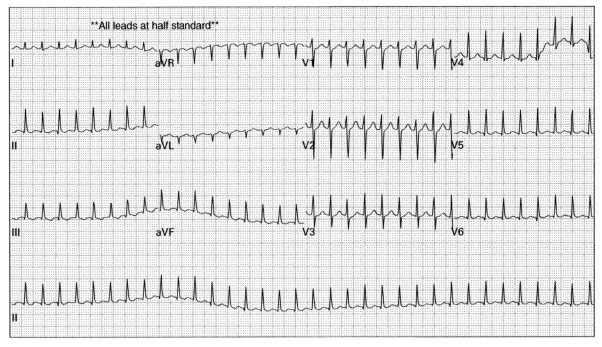

55. 23 year old man reports dyspnea and palpitations

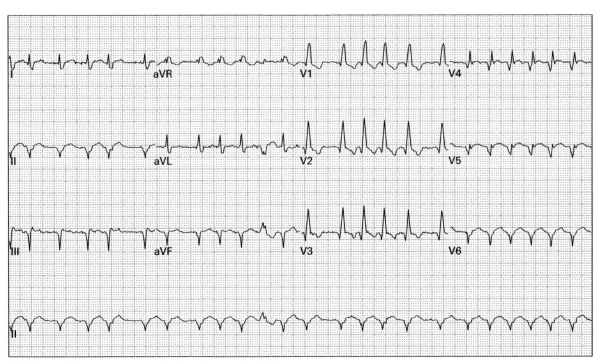

56. 57 year old man reports generalized weakness and palpitations

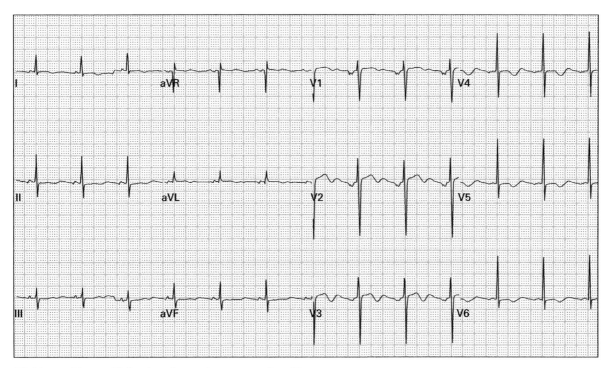

57. 54 year old man with five days of anorexia, nausea, and vomiting

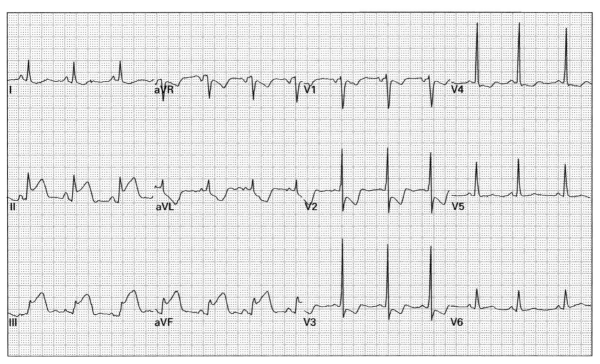

58. 66 year old woman with epigastric pain, nausea, dyspnea, and diaphoresis

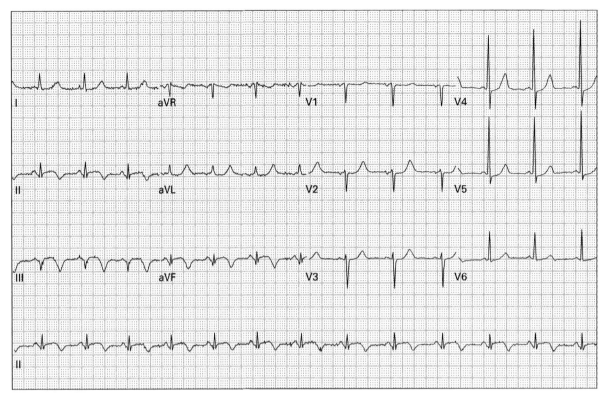

59. 70 year old woman with nine hours of chest pain and dyspnea

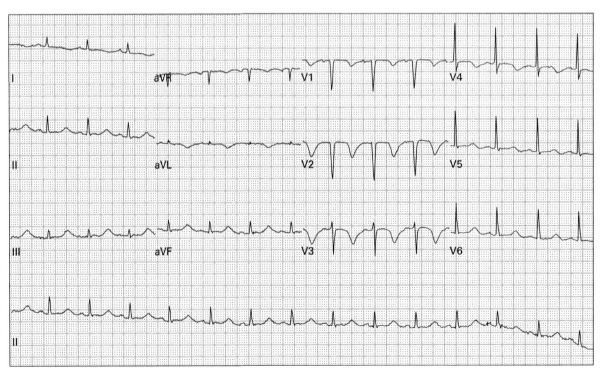

60. 52 year old alcoholic woman presents with frequent vomiting

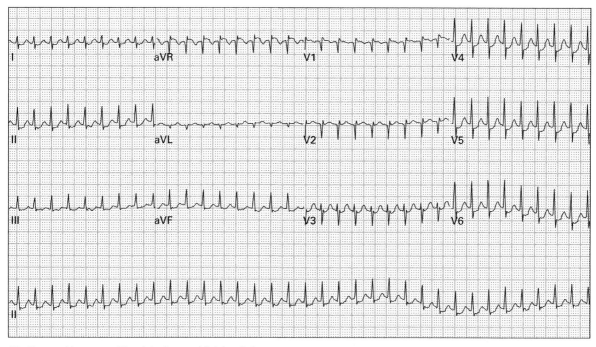

61. 45 year old woman with palpitations and lightheadedness

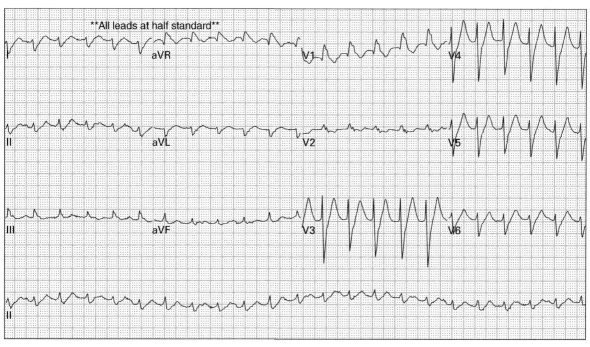

62. 45 year old man with severe lightheadedness

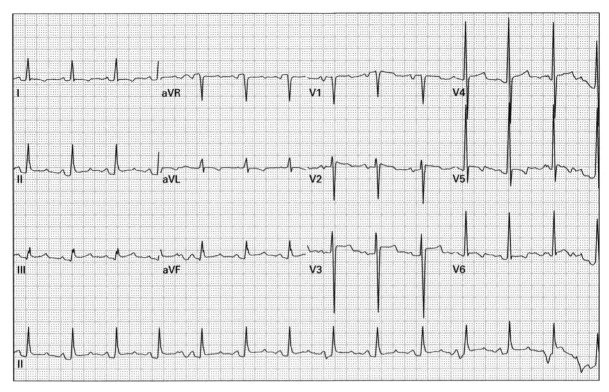

63. 52 year old man with sharp chest pain

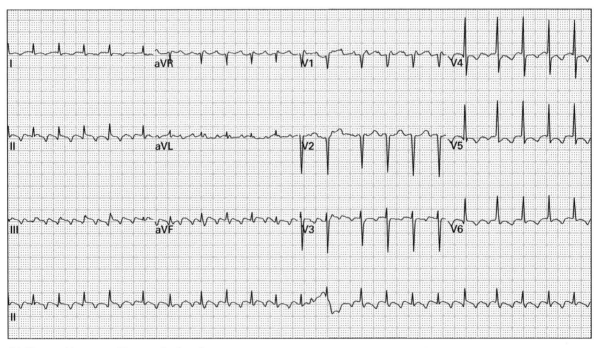

64. 71 year old woman with generalized weakness

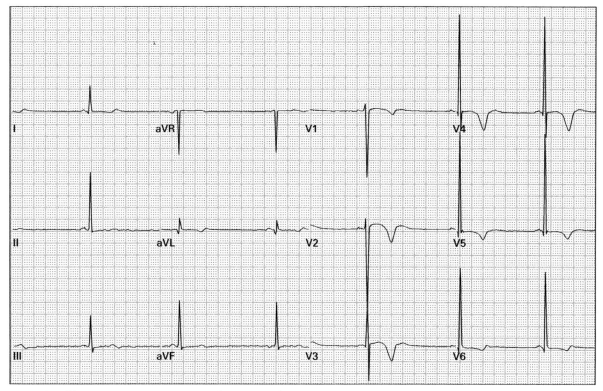

65. 34 year old woman presents unconscious with respiratory depression and pinpoint pupils

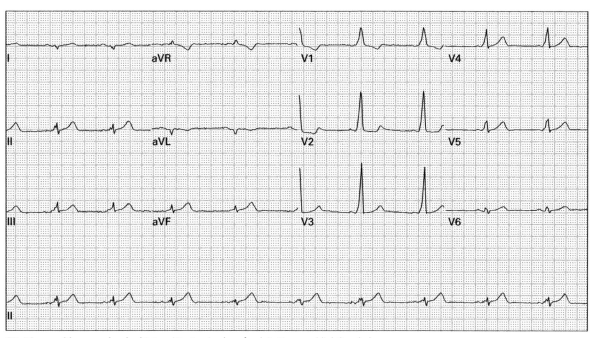

66. 36 year old woman has had intermittent episodes of palpitations and lightheadedness

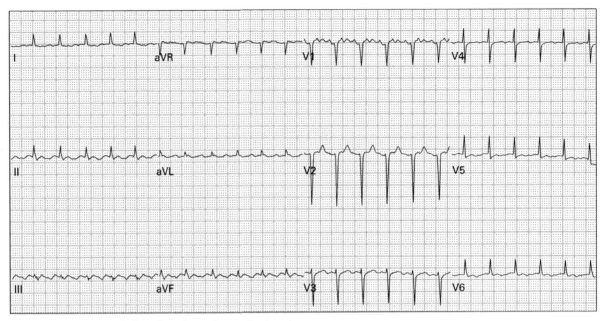

67. 70 year old woman with chest discomfort and generalized weakness

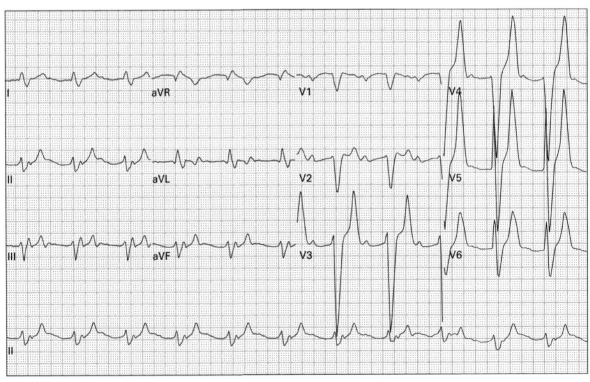

68. 41 year old man with end-stage renal failure presents with generalized weakness after missing his last three hemodialysis sessions

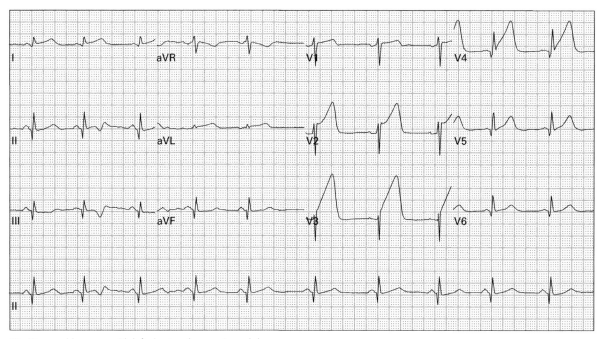

69. 45 year old woman with left chest and arm pain and dyspnea

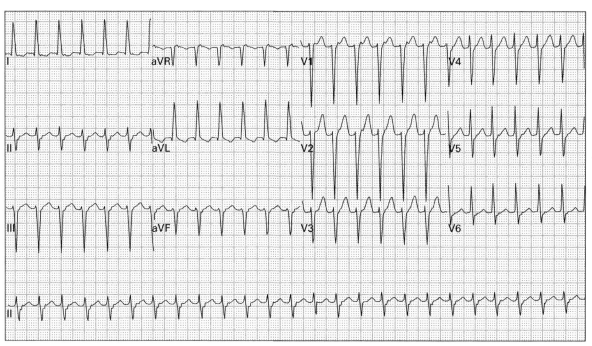

70. 78 year old woman with dyspnea and nausea

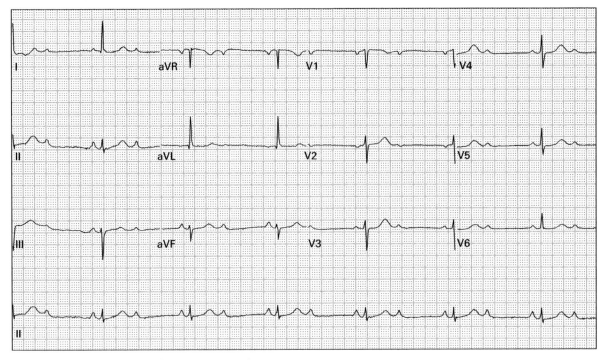

71. 75 year old woman presents after a syncopal episode

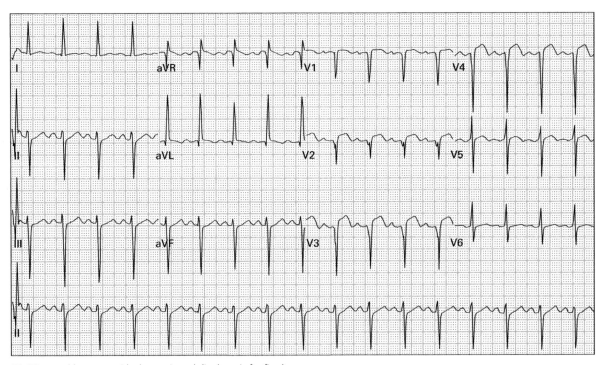

72. 50 year old woman with chest pain and diaphoresis for five hours

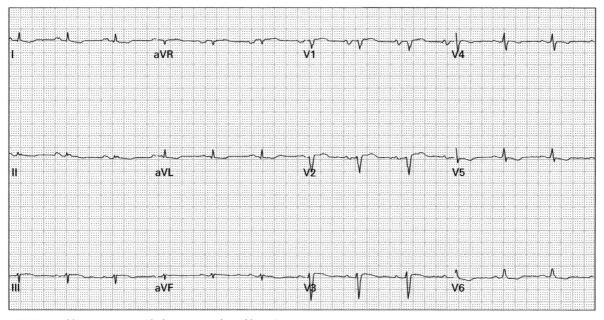

73. 59 year old man presents with dyspnea, cough, and hypoxia

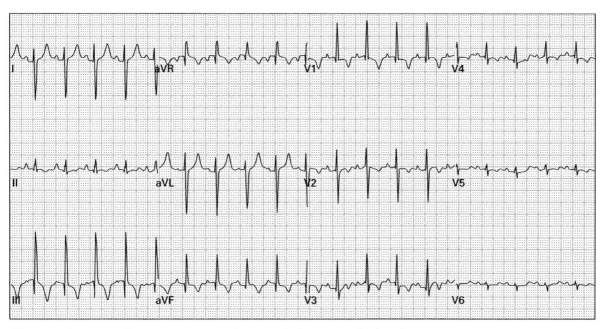

74. 62 year old woman with chest pain and severe dyspnea gradually worsening for three days

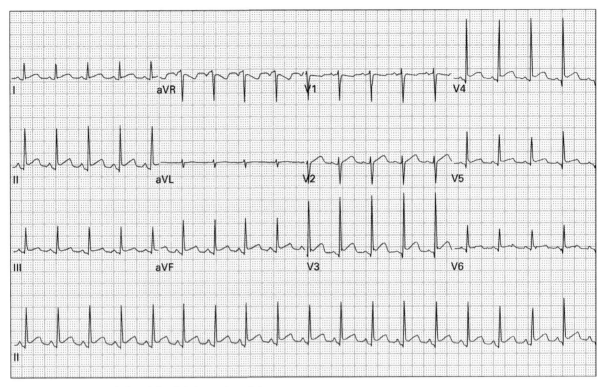

75. 40 year old man with sharp left-sided chest pain and dyspnea

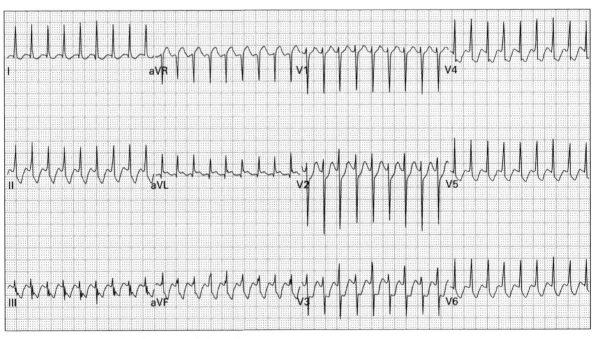

76. 28 year old woman with palpitations and chest pain

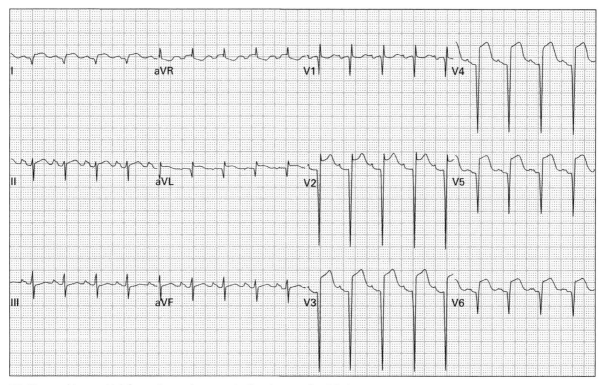

77. 53 year old man with left arm "squeezing sensation" and nausea for eight hours

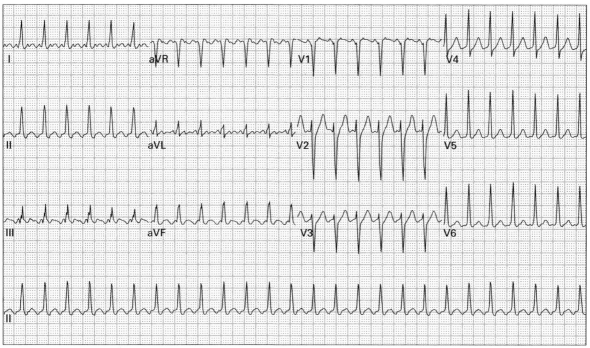

78. 69 year old woman with severe nausea and dyspnea

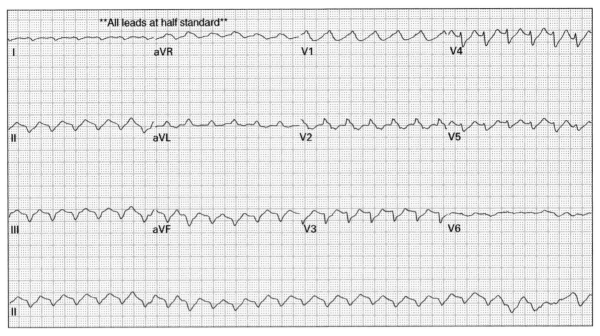

79. 68 year old man presents unconscious with blood pressure 108/60

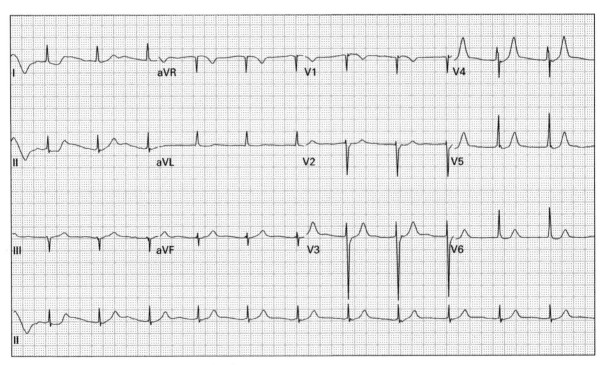

80. 65 year old woman with "funny feeling in chest"

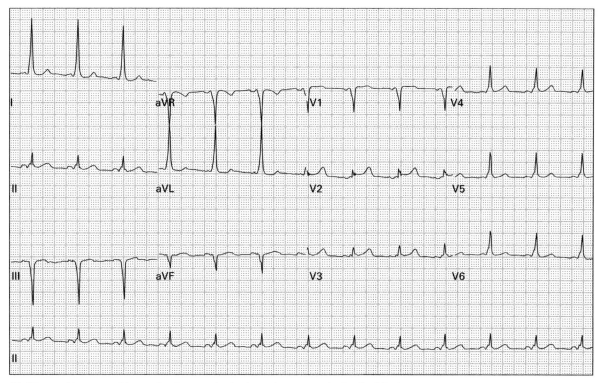

81. 55 year old woman with occasional syncopal episodes and a recent episode of palpitations

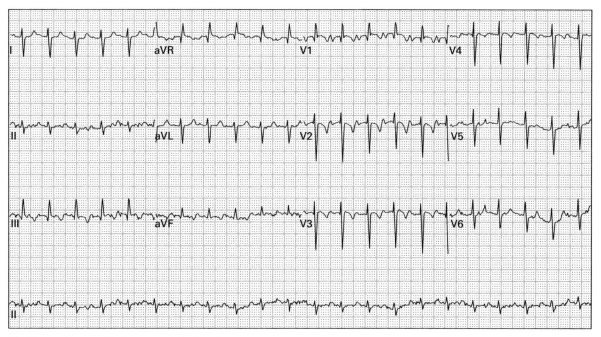

82. 69 year old man with dyspnea and diaphoresis

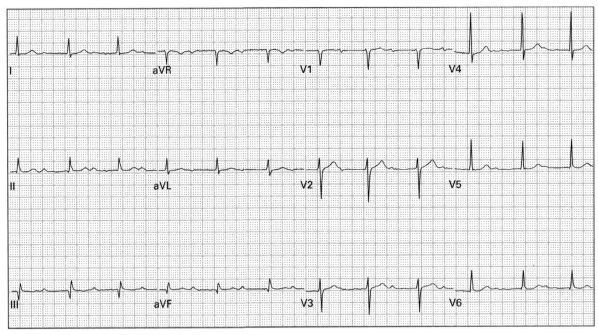

83. 79 year old man with abdominal pain

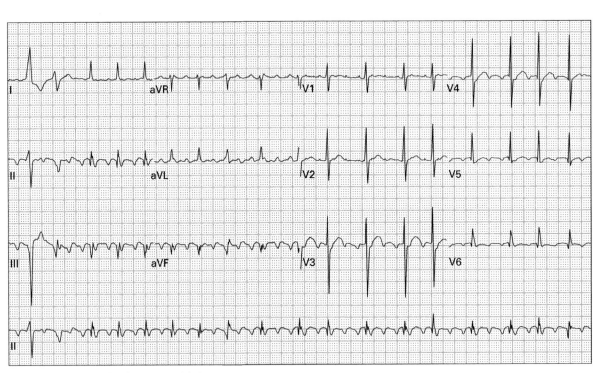

84. 85 year old man with palpitations and fatigue

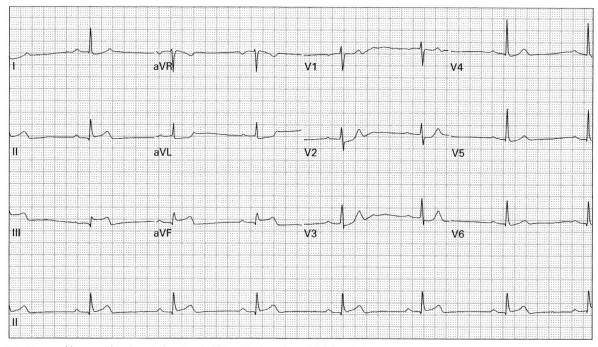

85. 63 year old man with epigastric burning, belching, diaphoresis, and lightheadedness

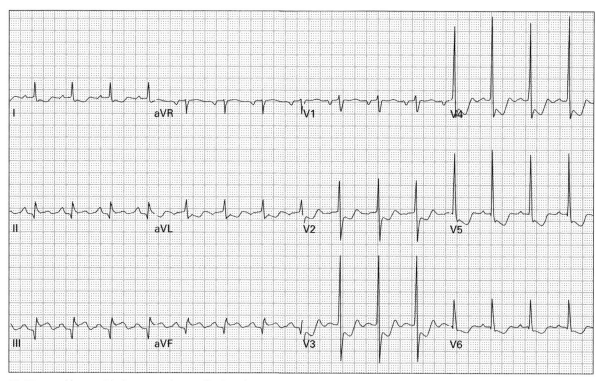

86. 70 year old man with dyspnea and generalized weakness

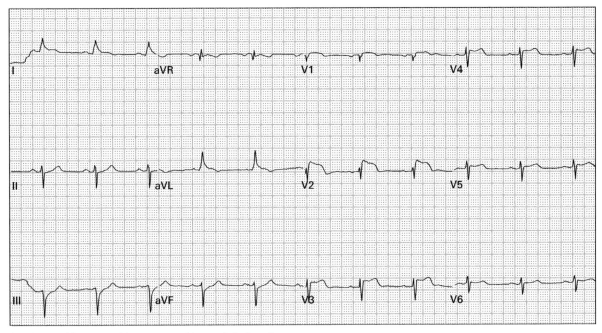

87. 70 year old woman with nausea, vomiting, and diaphoresis

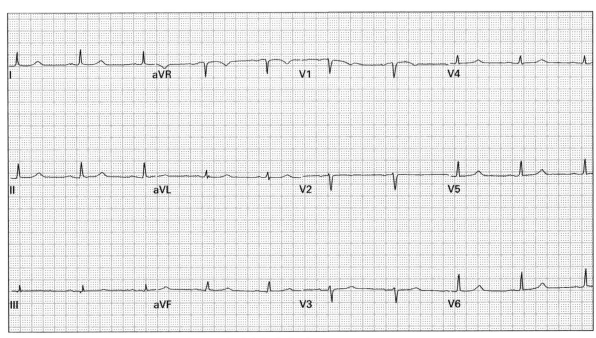

88. 55 year old morbidly obese woman with generalized abdominal pain

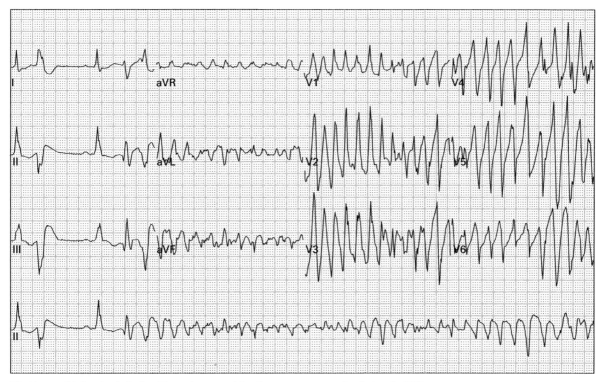

89. 44 year old chronic alcoholic with persistent vomiting; becomes unresponsive during the ECG

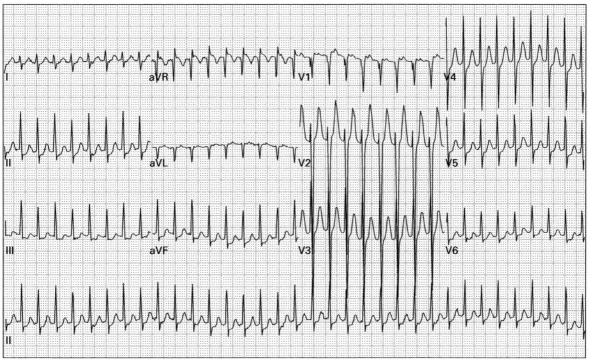

90. 25 year old woman with palpitations and lightheadedness

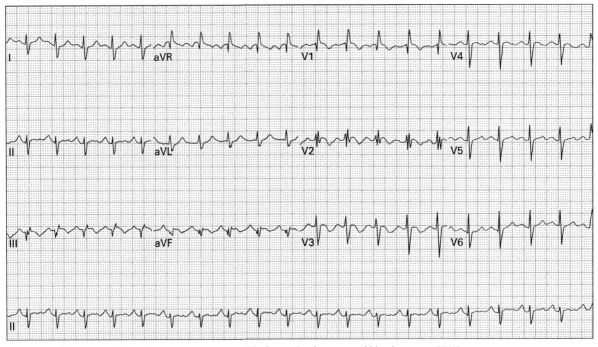

91. 28 year old woman eight weeks pregnant presents with chest pain, dyspnea, and blood pressure 80/40

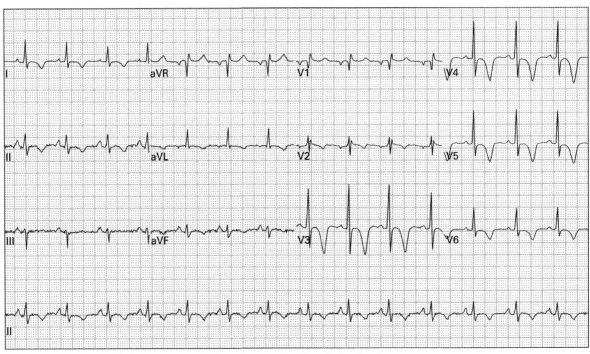

92. 47 year old woman with chest pain; now pain free after use of sublingual nitroglycerin

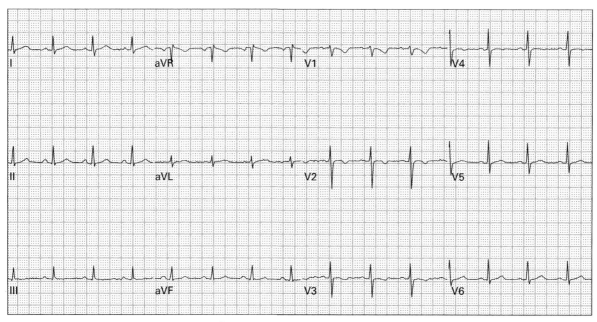

93. 38 year old woman with chest pain, dyspnea, fever, and productive cough

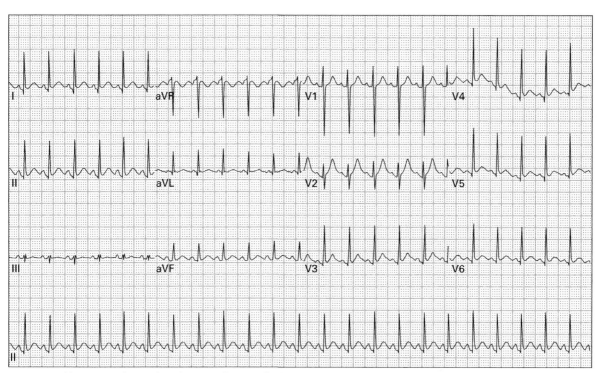

94. 46 year old woman with episodic palpitations, frequent diaphoresis, and a 15 pound weight loss over the past one month

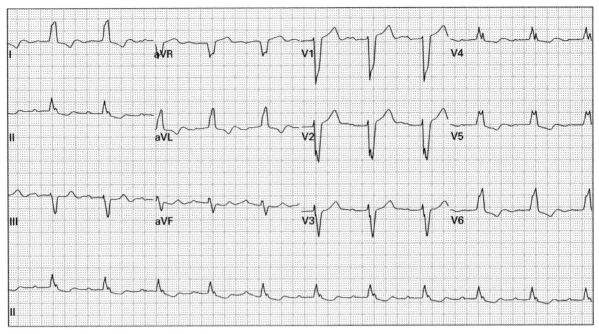

95. 84 year old woman with nausea and vomiting

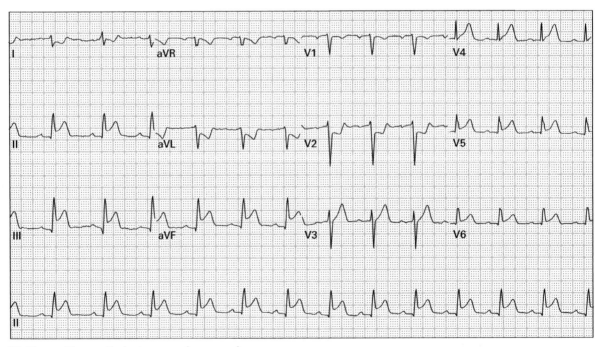

96. 57 year old man with chest pressure, dyspnea, and nausea

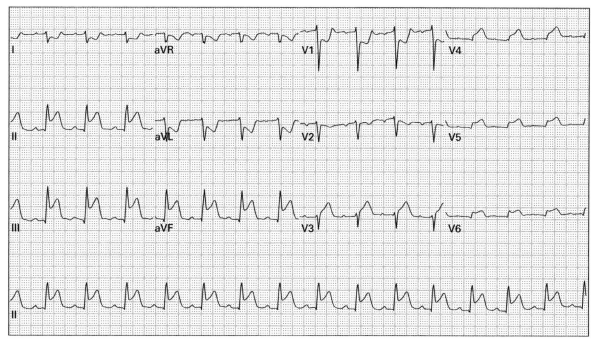

97. 57 year old man with chest pressure, dyspnea, and nausea (right-sided precordial leads)

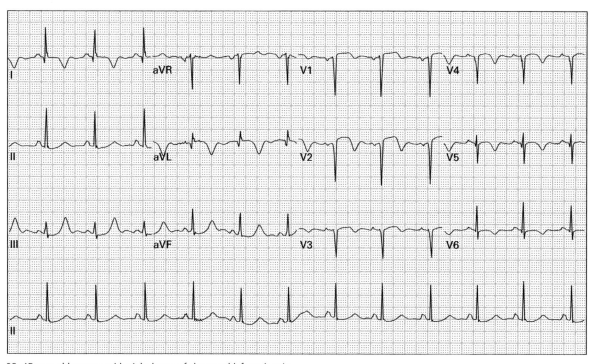

98. 45 year old woman with eight hours of chest and left neck pain

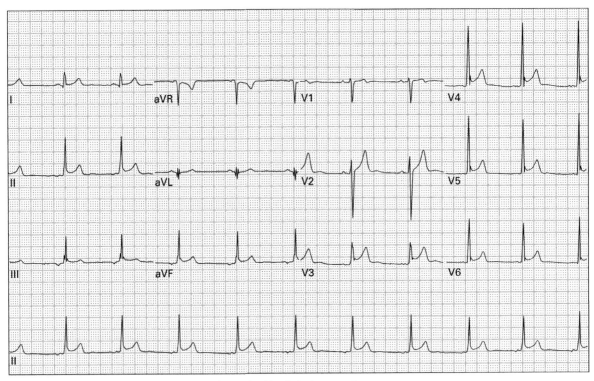

99. 24 year old woman had a syncopal episode after seeing blood; she has no pain

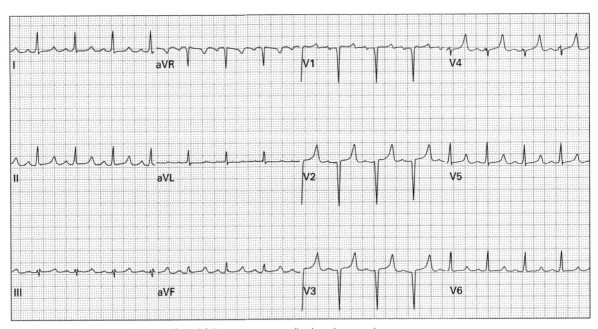

100. 26 year old woman with history of renal failure reports generalized weakness and nausea

ECG interpretations and comments

(Rates refer to ventricular rates unless otherwise specified; axis refers to QRS axis unless otherwise specified)

1. **Sinus rhythm (SR), rate 60, normal ECG.** SR is generally defined as having an atrial rate of 60–100/minute and a P-wave axis +15 to +75 degrees. Sinus beats can be identified by upright P-waves in leads I, II, III, and aVF; if the P-waves are inverted in any of these leads, it implies an ectopic atrial origin for the P-waves. The PR interval should be >0·20 seconds; a shorter PR interval suggests either an atrioventricular (AV) junctional origin or the presence of a pre-excitation syndrome (for example Wolff-Parkinson-White syndrome). The normal ECG often will demonstrate inverted T-waves in leads aVR and V1.

2. **SR with sinus arrhythmia, rate 66, benign early repolarization (BER).** Sinus arrhythmia is defined as sinus rhythm with slight variation (>0·16 seconds) in the sinus cycles. This produces mild irregularity in the rhythm and usually occurs at lower heart rates (<70/minute). BER is a normal variant often found in young healthy adults, especially men. Patients will have ST-segment elevation in many leads, although not in aVR or V1. The absence of reciprocal ST-segment changes helps distinguish this entity from acute myocardial infarction. Acute pericarditis can be difficult to distinguish from BER. The presence of PR-segment depression in various leads favors the diagnosis of acute pericarditis; however, the distinction between these two entities often must be made based on the patient history and physicial examination: acute pericarditis is classically associated with pleuritic sharp chest pain that changes with body position, and these patients may have a pericardial friction rub heard during cardiac auscultation.

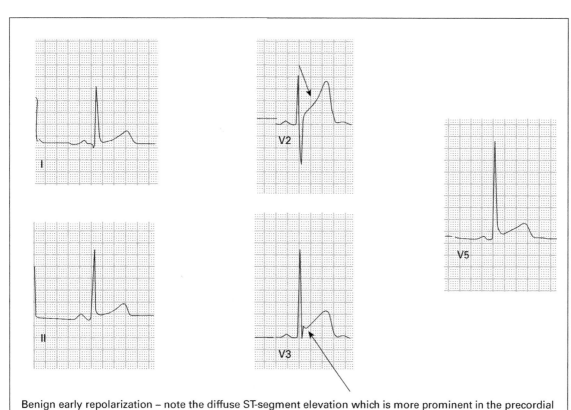

Benign early repolarization – note the diffuse ST-segment elevation which is more prominent in the precordial leads (leads V2, V3, and V5) when compared to the limb leads (I and II). The J point is elevated with elevation of the ST-segment maintaining the morphology of the ST-segment. The morphology of the elevated ST-segment is concave (large arrow), a feature which is highly suggestive of a non-AMI cause of ST-segment elevation. The J point is frequently notched or irregular (small arrow)

53

3. **SR, rate 91, with first degree AV block.** The normal PR-interval is 0·12–0·20 seconds. This patient has a marked first degree AV block with a PR-interval of 0·32 seconds.

4. **Ectopic atrial rhythm, rate 82, otherwise normal ECG.** P-waves in leads I, II, and aVF are inverted suggesting an ectopic origin of the atrial beats. The normal PR-interval (0·16 seconds) implies that the origin is in the atrium rather than in the AV junction.

5. **AV junctional rhythm, rate 50.** AV junctional rhythms are usually associated with a rate of 40–60/minute and narrow QRS complexes (unless there is a conduction abnormality, for example bundle branch block). If an AV junctional rhythm has a rate 61–100/minute, it is referred to as an "accelerated AV junctional rhythm;" if the rate is >100/minute, it is referred to as an "AV junctional tachycardia." In AV junctional rhythms, P-waves may be hidden or may precede or follow the QRS complex. When these "retrograde" P-waves precede the QRS, they will be associated with a short PR-interval (<0·12 seconds). This patient had recently started taking a calcium channel blocking medication for hypertension. When the medication was discontinued, SR returned and the ventricular rate increased.

6. **Accelerated idioventricular rhythm (AIVR), rate 65.** Ventricular escape rhythms are usually associated with rates 20–40/minute. When a ventricular rhythm is 40–110/minute, it is referred to as an "accelerated ventricular rhythm" or "accelerated idioventricular rhythm." When the rate exceeds 110/minute, "ventricular tachycardia" is diagnosed. This patient's rhythm strip demonstrates evidence of AV dissociation, easily seen in the latter portion of the strip. AIVR is commonly seen in the setting of AMI, especially after the administration of thrombolytic agents. AIVR is thought to be a marker of reperfusion. This patient's dysrhythmia resolved in minutes without therapy, typical of post-thrombolytic AIVR.

7. **SR, rate 100, right bundle branch block (RBBB).** RBBB is typically associated with an rSR' pattern in the right precordial leads, although a single, wide R-wave or a qR pattern may be seen instead. The S-wave in the lateral leads (I, aVL, V5, V6) is slightly wide, and the QRS duration is ≥0·12 seconds. If all the criteria are met except the QRS duration is ≤0·12 seconds, an incomplete RBBB is diagnosed. Leads V1–V3 often demonstrate ST-segment depression and inverted T-waves. Any ST-segment elevation should alert the healthcare provider to the possibility of AMI.

8. **SR, rate 80, first degree AV block, left bundle branch block (LBBB).** LBBB is characterized by prolonged QRS duration ≥0·12 seconds, leftward QRS axis, a broad monophasic R-wave in leads I and V6, and a deep wide S-wave in lead V1 (often times without any R-wave). The ST-segments and the T-waves are directed in an opposite direction to the main QRS vector in all leads (the rule of "appropriate discordance"). This patient had a pre-existing LBBB and borderline first degree AV block. The increased dose of the beta-receptor blocking medication caused a significant increase in the PR-interval. See figure on p. 55.

9. **SR, rate 81, left anterior fascicular block (LAFB).** LAFB is associated with a leftward QRS axis, a qR complex (small q-wave and large R-wave) or R-wave in leads I and aVL, rS complex (small r-wave and large S-wave) in lead III, and absence of other causes of leftward axis. The differential diagnosis of leftward axis includes the following: LAFB, LBBB, inferior myocardial infarction, left ventricular hypertrophy, ventricular ectopy, paced beats, and Wolff-Parkinson-White syndrome.

10. **SR, rate 85, RBBB, left posterior fascicular block (LPFB).** The combination of a RBBB plus a fascicular block is also called a "bifascicular block." LPFB is much less common than LAFB. It usually occurs concurrently with an RBBB rather than in isolation. The T-wave inversions in the inferior leads are commonly found with this type of bifascicular block. LPFB is associated with a rightward QRS axis, a qR complex (small q-wave and large R-wave) in lead III, and absence of other causes of rightward axis. The differential diagnosis of rightward axis includes the following: LPFB, lateral myocardial infarction, right ventricular hypertrophy, acute (for example pulmonary

This figure corresponds to case #8. LBBB pattern with appropriate ST-segment – T-wave changes

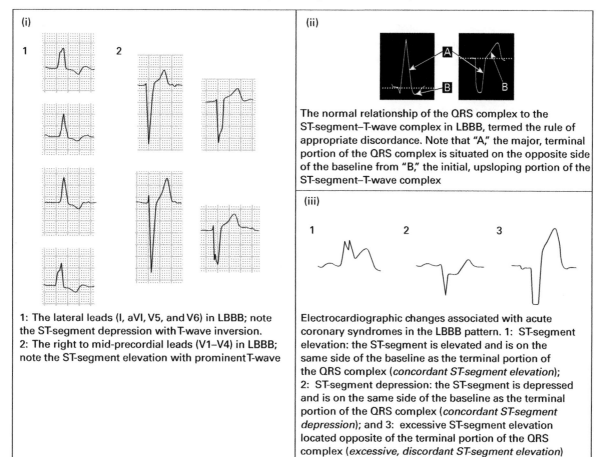

(i)

1: The lateral leads (I, aVl, V5, and V6) in LBBB; note the ST-segment depression with T-wave inversion.
2: The right to mid-precordial leads (V1–V4) in LBBB; note the ST-segment elevation with prominent T-wave

(ii)

The normal relationship of the QRS complex to the ST-segment–T-wave complex in LBBB, termed the rule of appropriate discordance. Note that "A," the major, terminal portion of the QRS complex is situated on the opposite side of the baseline from "B," the initial, upsloping portion of the ST-segment–T-wave complex

(iii)

Electrocardiographic changes associated with acute coronary syndromes in the LBBB pattern. 1: ST-segment elevation: the ST-segment is elevated and is on the same side of the baseline as the terminal portion of the QRS complex (*concordant ST-segment elevation*); 2: ST-segment depression: the ST-segment is depressed and is on the same side of the baseline as the terminal portion of the QRS complex (*concordant ST-segment depression*); and 3: excessive ST-segment elevation located opposite of the terminal portion of the QRS complex (*excessive, discordant ST-segment elevation*)

embolism) and chronic (for example emphysema) lung disease, ventricular ectopy, hyperkalemia, overdoses of sodium channel blocking drugs (for example cyclic antidepressants). Normal young or slender adults with a horizontally positioned heart can also demonstrate a rightward QRS axis on the ECG.

11. **AV junctional rhythm, rate 50, acute anterior and high lateral myocardial infarction.** P-waves are present with a short PR-interval (<0·12 seconds), suggesting an AV junctional origin of the beats. The rate is typical of an AV junctional origin. ST-segment elevation is present in the mid-precordial leads leading to the diagnosis of an anterior wall myocardial infarction (MI). ST-segment elevation is also present in leads I and aVL, corresponding to the high lateral wall of the left ventricle. Reciprocal ST-segment depression is present in the inferior leads. The presence of reciprocal changes significantly increases the specificity of ST-segment elevation for an acute MI.

12. **SR with second degree AV block type 1 (Mobitz I, Wenckebach), rate 50, left ventricular hypertrophy (LVH), RBBB.** Mobitz I is characterized by regular P-waves (the atrial rate here is approximately 65/minute) with progressive prolongation of the PR-interval until a P-wave fails to conduct to the ventricle. Usually there is also progressive shortening of the RR interval until the P-wave is non-conducted. LVH is diagnosed on this ECG based on the R-wave amplitude in lead aVL >11 mm. Leftward axis is due to LVH.

13. **Ventricular tachycardia (VT), rate 140.** When the ECG rhythm is a wide-complex regular tachycardia, the differential diagnosis includes sinus tachycardia (ST) with aberrant conduction, supraventricular tachycardia

(SVT) with aberrant conduction, and VT. ST is ruled out based on the absence of a regular association between atrial and ventricular complexes. The distinction between SVT with aberrant conduction versus VT is difficult. In this case, the presence of AV dissociation (P-waves are intermittently seen, especially in leads V1 and II) excludes the diagnosis of SVT. In general, wide-complex regular tachydysrhythmias that do not show regular sinus activity should always be treated as VT; inappropriate treatment of VT as an SVT may induce hemodynamic compromise.

14. **SR, rate 87, Wolff-Parkinson-White syndrome (WPW).** WPW, the most common ventricular pre-excitation syndrome, is characterized by the triad of:
    - short PR-interval <0·12 seconds
    - prolongation of the QRS complex >0·10 seconds
    - a slurred upstroke of the QRS complex ("delta wave").

    WPW can simulate ventricular hypertrophy, bundle branch block, and previous MI. Leftward axis in this case is attributed to WPW.

15. **ST, rate 155.** When the ECG rhythm is a narrow-complex regular tachycardia, the differential diagnosis includes ST, SVT, and atrial flutter. Distinguishing amongst these three entities is based on close evaluation of the atrial activity. In this case, there is a 1:1 relationship between the P-waves and the QRS complexes, thus confirming the diagnosis of ST.

16. **Sinus bradycardia (SB), rate 50, LVH, acute pericarditis.** LVH is diagnosed in this case based on the R-wave amplitude in V5 (or V6) + the S-wave amplitude in V1 >35 mm. Diffuse ST-segment elevation is also present. The absence of reciprocal ST-segment changes and the presence of (subtle) PR-segment depression in several leads favors the diagnosis of acute pericarditis rather than acute MI or BER. This patient's cardiac examination was notable for an audible friction rub.

17. **Atrial flutter with 2:1 AV conduction, rate 150.** The ECG rhythm is a narrow-complex regular tachycardia; therefore, the differential diagnosis is ST, SVT, and atrial flutter. Atrial activity ("flutter-waves") can be found in the inferior leads at a rate of 300/minute. The atrial complexes are inverted and manifest as a "sawtooth" pattern in the inferior leads, typical of atrial flutter. Whenever the ventricular rate is 150 ± 20/minute, atrial flutter should strongly be considered and the ECG should be closely scrutinized for the presence of flutter-waves.

18. **SR, rate 85, T-wave abnormality consistent with anterior and inferior ischemia, rightward axis.** The ECG is highly suggestive of acute pulmonary embolism, which this patient had. The ECG demonstrates the classic $S_I Q_{III} T_{III}$ finding (large S-wave in lead I, small Q-wave in lead III, inverted T-wave in lead III), present in 10–15% of cases of pulmonary embolism. T-wave inversions are common in pulmonary embolism, and the combination of T-wave inversions that occur simultaneously in the inferior and anteroseptal leads should strongly prompt consideration of this diagnosis. Rightward axis is often found on ECGs of patients with acute (for example acute pulmonary embolism) or chronic (for example emphysema) pulmonary disease.

19. **Atrial fibrillation with rapid ventricular response, rate 155.** When the ECG rhythm is a narrow-complex irregular tachycardia, the differential diagnosis includes atrial fibrillation, atrial flutter with variable AV conduction, and multifocal atrial tachycardia (MAT). Distinguishing between these three entities is based on close evaluation of the atrial activity. Atrial flutter will be associated with regular atrial activity (flutter-waves). MAT will be associated with irregular atrial activity, and the atrial complexes will vary in morphology (there must be at least three different morphologies for the diagnosis to be made). Atrial fibrillation will not be associated with any notable atrial complexes at all.

20. **AV sequential electronic pacemaker, rate 70, 100% capture.** Atrial pacing occurs, indicated by an initial pacemaker "spike" (PS). This is followed by an atrial complex, which then is followed by another PS after a

This figure corresponds to case #20. Atrioventricular paced dythm

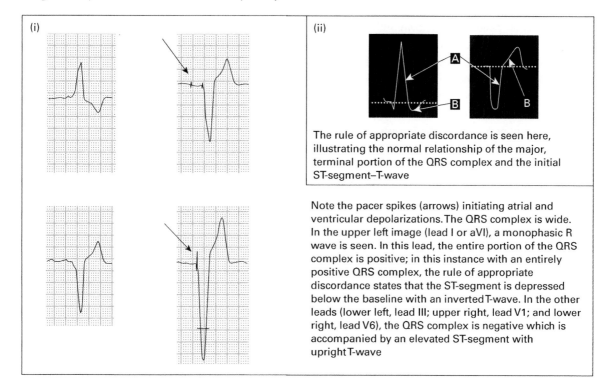

(i)

(ii)

The rule of appropriate discordance is seen here, illustrating the normal relationship of the major, terminal portion of the QRS complex and the initial ST-segment–T-wave

Note the pacer spikes (arrows) initiating atrial and ventricular depolarizations. The QRS complex is wide. In the upper left image (lead I or aVl), a monophasic R wave is seen. In this lead, the entire portion of the QRS complex is positive; in this instance with an entirely positive QRS complex, the rule of appropriate discordance states that the ST-segment is depressed below the baseline with an inverted T-wave. In the other leads (lower left, lead III; upper right, lead V1; and lower right, lead V6), the QRS complex is negative which is accompanied by an elevated ST-segment with upright T-wave

preset delay. The second PS is immediately followed by a QRS complex, indicating successful ventricular depolarization. The QRS complexes have an LBBB-type of morphology and ST-segment/T-wave discordance. The most important finding is that each pair of PSs is followed by ventricular "capture," indicating proper functioning of the electronic pacemaker.

21.   **AV junctional tachycardia, rate 110, RBBB.** P-waves preceding the QRS complexes are absent, thus excluding an atrial rhythm. In contrast, P-waves can be found **following** the QRS complexes (best seen in the precordial leads). This "retrograde" atrial activity is typical of AV junctional rhythms. An RBBB morphology of the QRS complexes is also noted. The rhythm converted to SR with RBBB after a single dose of intravenous adenosine.

22.   **ST, rate 110, RBBB, right ventricular hypertrophy (RVH), anteroseptal MI.** Although many criteria exist for the diagnosis of RVH, the most common are rightward axis, R:S ratio in lead V1 >1 and in V6 <1, and R-wave amplitude in lead V1 >7 mm. In the presence of RBBB, however, the R-wave amplitude in lead V1 must be >15 mm, as is the case here. This patient had developed RVH from severe chronic obstructive pulmonary disease. Q-waves are present in the right precordial leads, indicating an old anteroseptal MI.

23.   **Supraventricular tachycardia (SVT), rate 135, RBBB.** This wide-complex regular tachycardia without evidence of sinus P-waves should prompt immediate consideration of ventricular tachycardia. However, the treating physician was quickly able to obtain a copy of a previous ECG, (shown in case #7) which demonstrated sinus rhythm with a pre-existing RBBB. Most importantly, the QRS complex morphologies were identical between the two ECGs; therefore, the diagnosis of SVT with RBBB was made. The patient was treated successfully with adenosine.

24.   **Accelerated AV junctional rhythm, rate 84, prolonged QT, J-waves suggestive of hypothermia.** The artifact noted in the ECG was caused by shivering – this patient's body temperature was 25·6 degrees Celsius

(78·1 degrees Fahrenheit). J-waves (also known as "Osborne waves") are most notable in the precordial leads. These are positive deflections in the terminal portions of the QRS complex. The exact cause of the J-wave in hypothermic patients is unknown. Although considered highly sensitive and specific for hypothermia, J-waves are not pathognomonic for hypothermia. Hypothermia is also associated with prolongation of the QRS and QT-intervals (QT = 0·540 seconds in this case; QTc = 0·640 seconds). Other causes of prolonged QT-interval include hypokalemia, hypomagnesemia, hypocalcemia, acute myocardial ischemia, elevated intracranial pressure, drugs with sodium channel blocking effects (for example cyclic antidepressants, quinidine, etc.), and congenital prolonged QT syndrome. QT-interval prolongation in hypothermia and hypocalcemia is completely due to ST-segment prolongation; the T-waves remain unchanged. This is not true for other causes of QT prolongation.

25. **SR, rate 66, occasional premature atrial complexes, LVH, previous high-lateral MI, non-specific T-wave abnormality in inferior leads, digoxin effect.** The second and the seventh QRS complexes occur early in the cycle and are preceded by subtle P-waves; therefore these are considered premature atrial contractions (PACs). Q-waves present in leads I and aVL occur due to a previous MI involving the lateral wall of the left ventricle. When leads I and aVL are the only lateral leads involved, it is presumed to involve the "high lateral" portion of the left ventricle. The ST-segment depression/T-wave inversions in leads V5 and V6 have an appearance similar to the end of a hockey stick. This "hockey stick" appearance is often associated with digoxin use (referred to as "digoxin effect"). It is **not** necessarily associated with digoxin toxicity, however. PACs are also a common finding in patients who take digoxin.

26. **Electronic ventricular pacemaker, rate 80, 100% capture.** The ST-segments and T-waves are "appropriately discordant" to the QRS complexes, similar to LBBB.

27. **SVT, rate 165.** The rhythm is a narrow-complex regular tachycardia. The distinction between the three main causes (ST, SVT, and atrial flutter) is made based on the presence and type of atrial activity. In this case, retrograde P-waves are seen in the inferior leads, a common finding in SVT. This patient converted to SR with vagal maneuvers.

This figure corresponds to case #29. Prominent T-waves of BER

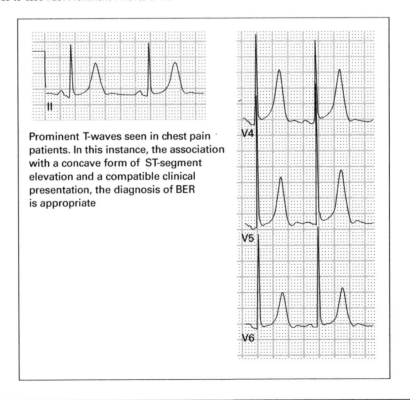

Prominent T-waves seen in chest pain patients. In this instance, the association with a concave form of ST-segment elevation and a compatible clinical presentation, the diagnosis of BER is appropriate

28. **SR with sinus arrhythmia, rate 75, persistent juvenile T-wave pattern.** Normal children and adolescents have a slight posterior orientation of the T-waves, producing inversions in the right precordial leads. With advancing age the T-wave orientation becomes more anterior, producing upright T-waves in leads V2–V3 and sometimes in lead V1 as well. Normal young adults (≤40 years of age), especially women, may have a persistence of the T-wave inversions in leads V1–V3. This is referred to as a "persistent juvenile T-wave pattern." These T-wave inversions are asymmetric and shallow. If the inversions are symmetric or deep, or if the patient is >45–50 years of age, myocardial ischemia should be assumed.

These figures correspond to case #30. Inferolateroposterior AMI with right ventricular acute infarction

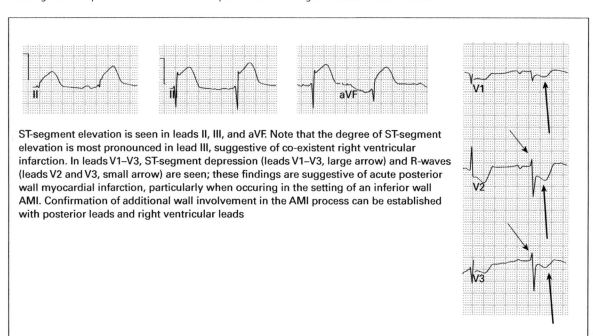

ST-segment elevation is seen in leads II, III, and aVF. Note that the degree of ST-segment elevation is most pronounced in lead III, suggestive of co-existent right ventricular infarction. In leads V1–V3, ST-segment depression (leads V1–V3, large arrow) and R-waves (leads V2 and V3, small arrow) are seen; these findings are suggestive of acute posterior wall myocardial infarction, particularly when occuring in the setting of an inferior wall AMI. Confirmation of additional wall involvement in the AMI process can be established with posterior leads and right ventricular leads

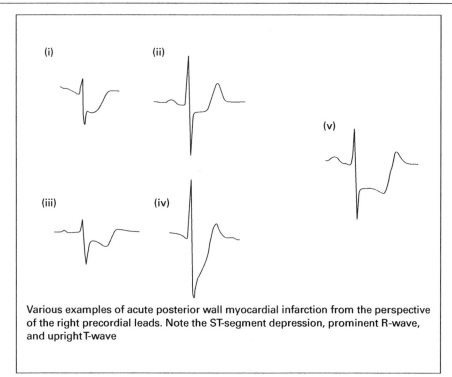

Various examples of acute posterior wall myocardial infarction from the perspective of the right precordial leads. Note the ST-segment depression, prominent R-wave, and upright T-wave

This figure refers to case #31. Right-sided chest leads with right ventricular and posterior AMI

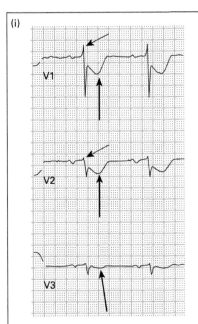

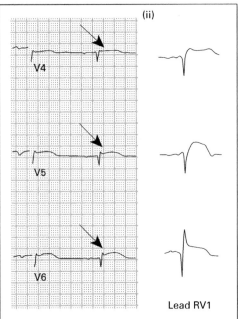

Lead RV1

Right-sided chest leads V1–V6 demonstrate findings consistent with acute posterior wall AMI and right ventricular (RV) infraction. Note the R-waves (small arrows) in right leads V1 and V2 associated with ST-segment depression and T-wave inversion (large arrows) in right leads V1–V3; these findings are consistent with posterior wall AMI. The ST-segment depression (arrow head) in right leads V4–V6 is indicative of an acute RV myocardial infarction; the clinician is reminded that the magnitude of ST-segment depression is frequently minimal in the RV infarction patient because of the relatively small size of the RV myocardial muscle mass (less myocardium produces less of a current of injury and, therefore, ST-segment elevation of lesser magnitude)

Additional examples of ST-segment elevation in lead RV4, indicative of an acute RV myocardial infarction. Single lead RV4 (placed in similar position to lead V4 yet on the right chest) is equal to an entire array of right-sided leads RV1–RV6 in detecting RV infarction

29. **SR with sinus arrhythmia, rate 65, LVH, BER.** The most notable characteristic in this ECG is the presence of prominent T-waves. These may be an early finding in acute myocardial ischemia, but prominent T-waves may be found in other conditions as well, including hyperkalemia, acute pericarditis, LVH, BER, bundle branch block, and pre-excitation syndromes. This patient had serial ECGs that showed no changes with time, and her workup for cardiac ischemia proved negative. See figure on p. 58.

30. **SR with first degree AV block, rate 62, acute inferolateral MI, possible right ventricular (RV) MI.** ST-segment elevation is present in the inferior and lateral leads with reciprocal ST-segment depression in leads I, aVL, and V1–V3. When the magnitude of ST-segment elevation in lead III exceeds that found in lead II, RV infarction is likely. A more definitive diagnosis of RV MI can be made using right-sided precordial leads (see ECG #31). See figures on p. 59.

31. **Right-sided precordial leads (same patient as in case #30): SR with first degree AV block, rate 62, acute inferior and RV MI.** The diagnosis of acute RV MI is confirmed by the presence of ST-segment elevation

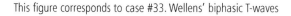

This figure corresponds to case #33. Wellens' biphasic T-waves

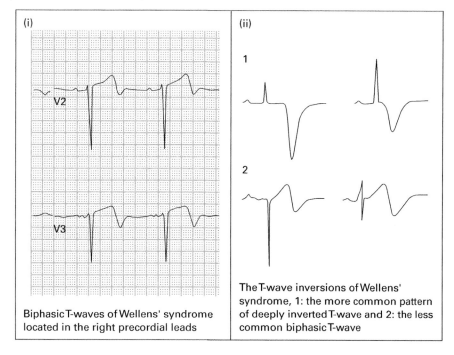

Biphasic T-waves of Wellens' syndrome located in the right precordial leads

The T-wave inversions of Wellens' syndrome, 1: the more common pattern of deeply inverted T-wave and 2: the less common biphasic T-wave

in any of the lateral right precordial leads (V4R, V5R, or V6R). A "right-sided ECG" involves placing the precordial ECG leads across the right side of the chest in mirror image to the normal ECG. The limb leads remain in an unchanged position. Acute RV infarction occurs in approximately one-third of patients with acute inferior MI and is associated with increased morbidity and mortality. In the emergency setting, the diagnosis of RV MI is important because it mandates cautious use of nitrates and other preload reducing agents; otherwise, profound hypotension may occur.

32. **SR, rate 75, frequent premature ventricular contractions (PVCs) in a pattern of bigeminy ("ventricular bigeminy").** Strokes, either ischemic or hemorrhagic, are often associated with changes on the ECG. Tachydysrhythmias, AV blocks, ST-segment changes, and T-wave abnormalities have been reported with strokes; the findings are usually transient, as was the case with this patient.

33. **SR, rate 70, acute inferior and anterolateral MI with T-wave abnormality consistent with ongoing ischemia.** The presence of Q-waves in the inferior, anterior, and lateral leads indicates completed infarction in these areas. There are also biphasic T-waves in the anterior leads (V2–V4) and inverted T-waves in the lateral leads (V5–V6, I, aVL) suggesting persistent ischemia in uninfarcted myocardium. The biphasic T-wave pattern in the mid-precordial leads was described in 1982 by Wellens and colleagues[1] as being highly specific for a large proximal left anterior descending artery (LAD) obstructive lesion. The lesion is best treated with percutaneous coronary intervention (angioplasty or stent placement); it does not respond well to medical management. This biphasic T-wave pattern, which has come to be known as "Wellens' sign," may persist or even develop when the patient is not experiencing pain. This patient had urgent coronary angiography which demonstrated 90% obstruction in the proximal LAD. He was successfully treated with angioplasty.

34. **SR with frequent premature atrial complexes (PACs) in a pattern of atrial trigeminy, rate 61.** The rhythm is regularly irregular because of the occurrence of PACs. PACs are identified when P-waves occur early in the rhythm. The morphology of the P-waves are often slightly different to the sinus P-waves, and the PR-interval may be slightly different as well. PACs cause the sinus node to reset, leading to a pause in the rhythm before the next sinus beat occurs.

35. **AV junctional rhythm, rate 40, LVH, septal MI, T-wave abnormality consistent with inferior and anterolateral ischemia.** P-waves are absent for most of the ECG and the QRS complexes are narrow; therefore, a junctional rhythm is diagnosed. A single P-wave is found immediately preceding the final QRS complex on the rhythm strip, but is unlikely to have been conducted because the very short PR-interval. Q-waves are found in leads V1–V2 consistent with a prior MI. Inverted T-waves in the inferior and anterolateral leads indicate acute ischemia (probably due to the bradycardia). This patient was treated with glucagon for beta-blocker toxicity, after which SR returned, the heart rate increased to 70, and the T-wave inversions all resolved.

36. **Atrial flutter with variable block, rate 167.** The rhythm is a narrow-complex irregular tachycardia. The differential diagnosis includes atrial fibrillation, atrial flutter with variable block, and multifocal atrial tachycardia. Distinguishing between these three dysrhythmias requires close inspection of the ECG for evidence of atrial activity. In this case, inverted flutter-waves are found in the inferior leads, confirming the diagnosis of atrial flutter. The rhythm is irregular because there exist varying degrees of AV block (2:1, 3:1, and 4:1). ST-segment depressions are found in the lateral leads. This is a common finding in tachydysrhythmias, especially SVT, and does **not** necessarily indicate a critical coronary stenosis. Electrical alternans (varying amplitudes of every second QRS complex) is present in leads V5 and V6. In the patient in SR, electrical alternans (EA) suggests the presence of a pericardial effusion. However, EA is not an uncommon finding in tachydysrhythmias and has no clinical significance.

37. **SR, rate 69, acute inferolateral MI.** ST-segment depression in leads aVL and V1–V3 is typical of the reciprocal changes associated with acute inferior MI.

38. **Atrial fibrillation with rapid ventricular response, rate 127, bifascicular block (RBBB + LAFB).** When the ECG rhythm is a wide-complex irregular tachycardia, the differential diagnosis includes atrial fibrillation with aberrant conduction (for example bundle branch block), atrial fibrillation with WPW, and polymorphic ventricular tachycardia (PVT). The distinction between these entities can be made by closely evaluating the rate and QRS morphologies. Atrial fibrillation with aberrant conduction usually will not exceed a ventricular rate of 200/minute, in contrast to the other two dysrhythmias, which usually are associated with ventricular rates in excess of 200–250/minute. Additionally, the morphology of the QRS complexes remains unchanged on the ECG in atrial fibrillation with aberrant conduction, whereas both atrial fibrillation with WPW and PVT will demonstrate significant variation in the width and amplitudes of the QRS complexes. The distinction between atrial fibrillation with WPW and PVT is often more difficult. PVT, however, tends to have a more chaotic appearance and patients are almost always profoundly unstable. In either case, when rates exceed 250/minute, patients are likely to decompensate rapidly and emergent cardioversion is the safest treatment. RBBB is diagnosed here by the usual criteria – rsR pattern in V1, QRS ≥0·12 seconds, wide S-wave in the lateral leads. LAFB is diagnosed based on the leftward axis (absent any other causes of leftward axis), qR pattern in aVL, and rS pattern in III.

39. **VT, rate 170.** The ECG could easily be mistaken for SVT with RBBB based on the QRS complex morphology in lead V1 and the appearance of retrograde P-waves following the QRS complexes. However, it is important to remember that VT can simulate either an RBBB or an LBBB pattern, and it can also be associated with retrograde P-waves. The patient had repetitive episodes of this dysrhythmia despite medical treatment. Ablative therapy was curative. In the electrophysiology laboratory, this was confirmed to be VT. See figure on p. 63.

40. **SR with occasional PACs, rate 80, LVH, acute inferior MI with posterior extension.** Posterior MI (PMI) usually occurs in association with inferior MI, less often in association with lateral MI, and rarely (<5%) in isolation. Normally, acute ischemia and infarction are associated with ST-segment elevation, T-wave inversions, and development of Q-waves. Because the standard precordial ECG leads (primarily leads V1–V3) provide an "inverted" image of the posterior portion of the heart, acute PMI will be associated with "inverted findings" in those same leads. In other words, acute PMI will produce ST-segment depression, large upright T-waves, and progressive development of large R-waves in leads V1–V3 as is seen in this case. Another method of detecting

This figure corresponds to case #39. Wide complex tachycardia consistent with ventricular tachycardia – numerous features in the wide complex tachycardia presentation which suggest ventricular tachycardia

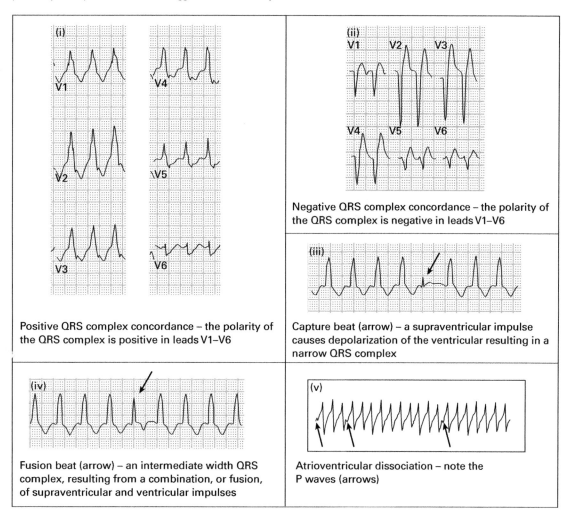

(i)
V1
V4
V2
V5
V3
V6

Positive QRS complex concordance – the polarity of the QRS complex is positive in leads V1–V6

(ii)
V1   V2   V3
V4   V5   V6

Negative QRS complex concordance – the polarity of the QRS complex is negative in leads V1–V6

(iii)

Capture beat (arrow) – a supraventricular impulse causes depolarization of the ventricular resulting in a narrow QRS complex

(iv)

Fusion beat (arrow) – an intermediate width QRS complex, resulting from a combination, or fusion, of supraventricular and ventricular impulses

(v)

Atrioventricular dissociation – note the P waves (arrows)

acute PMI is to perform an ECG with "posterior leads" (using the standard ECG, simply place leads V5 and V6 on the left back just inferolateral and inferomedial to the inferior pole of the scapula) and evaluating for the standard ST-segment elevation, T-wave inversions, and Q-waves. In this case, lead V6 was placed inferolateral to the inferior pole of the scapula. Slight ST-segment elevation is noted, confirming acute PMI.

41.   **SR, rate 70, acute inferior and PMI.** This ECG is from the same patient as in case #40, approximately two hours later. The patient had persistent pain despite thrombolytic and other medical therapy. The current ECG demonstrates development of Q-waves in the inferior leads and persistent ST-segment elevation, indicating ongoing ischemia. The ECG also demonstrates enlargement of the R-waves in the right precordial leads, indicative of PMI. A short time later, the patient underwent successful angioplasty and stent placement.

42.   **SB with second degree AV block type 2 (Mobitz II), rate 50, LBBB.** Mobitz II AV conduction is characterized by intermittent non-conducted P-waves, similar to Mobitz I. However, in contrast to Mobitz I, Mobitz II is associated with constant PR-intervals in those beats that are conducted. Mobitz II is usually associated with a bundle branch block.

43. **SR, rate 88, first degree AV block, previous inferior MI.** The rhythm could easily be misdiagnosed as an accelerated AV junctional rhythm because P-waves are not well-seen in most leads, including the lead II rhythm strip. However, lead V1 **does** show regular P-waves with a marked first degree AV block. P-waves are obscured by ("buried in") the T-waves in other leads. The T-waves in leads V2–V4 are actually slightly deformed by the buried P-wave. When a 12-lead ECG is obtained, **all** of the leads must be carefully studied to diagnose the underlying rhythm, not just the lead II rhythm strip. In many instances, V1 instead will be the best lead to identify P-waves.

44. **SR, rate 72, previous septal MI, inferior and anterolateral ischemia, prolonged QT.** The septal Q-waves and the diffuse T-wave inversions in this case were chronic. However, the QT-interval prolongation (QT = 0·516 seconds, QTc = 0·565 seconds) was new. The prolonged QT and the carpopedal spasm were due to hypocalcemia (5·0 mg/dL; normal = 8·8–10·2 mg/dL). Other common electrolyte-related causes of prolonged QT are hypokalemia and hypomagnesemia. In contrast to most other causes, the prolonged QT-interval in hypocalcemia is completely due to prolongation of the ST-segment; the duration of the T-wave remains unchanged. This is also true for hypothermia.

45. **SR, rate 95, poor R-wave progression (PRWP), T-wave abnormality consistent with inferior and anterolateral ischemia, prolonged QT.** PRWP is defined when the R-wave amplitude in lead V3 ≤3 mm. This finding is suggestive of a previous anteroseptal MI, but it may also be caused by LVH, abnormally high placement of the mid-precordial electrodes, or it may simply occur as a normal variant. The diffuse T-wave inversions in this case were new. The prolonged QT-interval (QT = 0·448 seconds, QTc = 0·560 seconds) in this case was due to acute myocardial ischemia. Note that the prolonged QT-interval here is caused by a widened T-wave, in contrast to case #44 where the prolonged QT-interval was caused by ST-segment prolongation. See figure on p. 65.

46. **ST, rate 155, T-wave abnormality consistent with anterolateral ischemia.** The main diagnostic considerations in a narrow-complex tachycardia are ST, SVT, and atrial flutter. P-waves precede every QRS-complex with a normal PR-interval, thus ruling out SVT. Close evaluation fails to disclose any flutter-waves, thus ruling out atrial flutter. There is an isolated Q-wave in lead III. Isolated Q-waves occasionally occur in lead III or aVF and do not have any clinical relevance. T-wave inversions in the lateral leads were new. The nausea and vomiting were this patient's "anginal equivalent." The protracted course of the nausea and vomiting induced dehydration and tachycardia.

47. **SR, dual chamber electronic pacemaker, rate 80, 100% capture.** This type of pacemaker produces an atrial impulse if native atrial activity does not occur. In this case, the patient's sinus node appears to be functioning properly. The ventricular stimulus occurs in response to the atrial output, whether it is an electronic or native stimulus.

48. **Atrial fibrillation with rapid ventricular response, rate 150, LAFB.** The narrow-complex irregular rhythm should prompt consideration of atrial flutter with variable block and MAT in addition to atrial fibrillation. However, the absence of any well-defined atrial activity rules out atrial flutter and MAT.

49. **Atrial flutter with variable block, rate 84, previous septal MI, T-wave abnormality consistent with lateral ischemia.** Flutter-waves are noted in the inferior leads, although somewhat more subtle than in previous examples. In this case, lead V1 provides the best "view" of atrial activity. Buried P-waves cause the T-waves to exhibit an increased amplitude or a slightly deformed appearance in lead V1.

50. **SR, rate 75, acute lateral MI.** Reciprocal ST-segment depression is present in the inferior and anteroseptal leads. Q-waves have already begun to develop indicating completed infarction of some myocardial tissue. However, the presence of persistent ST-segment elevation indicates that there is still viable myocardium that is acutely ischemic and salvageable.

This figure corresponds to case #45. Anterior wall T-wave inversions consistent with ischemia

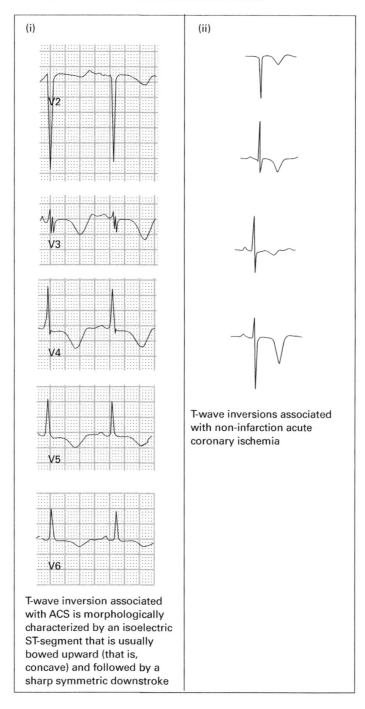

(i)

(ii)

T-wave inversions associated with non-infarction acute coronary ischemia

T-wave inversion associated with ACS is morphologically characterized by an isoelectric ST-segment that is usually bowed upward (that is, concave) and followed by a sharp symmetric downstroke

51.   **SR, rate 52, T-wave abnormality consistent with anteroseptal ischemia.** These T-wave inversions in leads V1–V3 should not be assumed to be persistent juvenile T-waves, a normal variant (see case #28), because they are symmetric and because the patient is >50 years of age. An isolated Q-wave in lead III is of no clinical significance. The T-wave inversions in this case were the result of a prior non-Q-wave MI. Pulmonary embolism

should also be considered when T-wave inversions are found in the right precordial leads. Her workup did not show evidence of acute ischemia or pulmonary embolism.

52. **SR with first degree AV block, rate 80, non-specific intraventricular conduction delay and peaked T-waves suggestive of hyperkalemia.** T-waves associated with hyperkalemia are typically abnormally large and, unlike other causes of prominent T-waves (acute myocardial ischemia, acute pericarditis, LVH, BER, bundle branch block, and pre-excitation syndromes), they tend to be peaked and narrow-based. Peaked T-waves are the earliest finding in hyperkalemia. Their appearance does not correlate with specific serum potassium levels. As potassium levels rise, other ECG abnormalities develop including P-wave flattening, PR-interval and QRS prolongation (intraventricular conduction delay), high-grade AV blocks, intraventricular conduction abnormalities (including fascicular blocks and bundle branch blocks), and finally a sine-wave appearance of the rhythm. The appearance of these various abnormalities does not correlate well with specific serum potassium levels. This patient's serum potassium level was 9·1 mEq/L (normal 3·5–5·3 mEq/L).

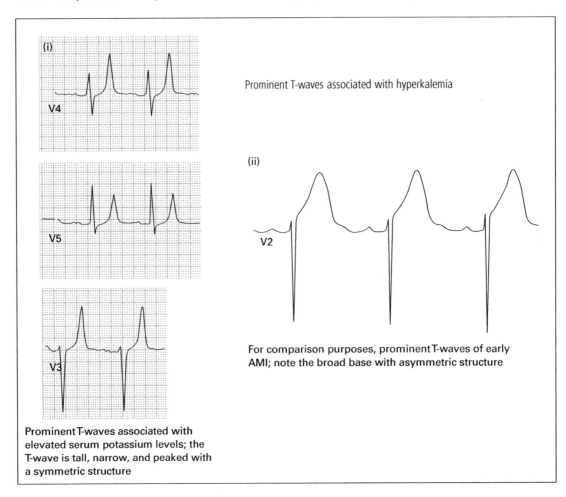

Prominent T-waves associated with hyperkalemia

(ii)

For comparison purposes, prominent T-waves of early AMI; note the broad base with asymmetric structure

Prominent T-waves associated with elevated serum potassium levels; the T-wave is tall, narrow, and peaked with a symmetric structure

53. **Atrial flutter with 2:1 AV conduction, rate 150.** The ventricular rate of 150/minute should prompt a search for flutter-waves. In this case, they **are** found in the inferior leads and produce the classic "sawtooth pattern," especially in lead II. Upright atrial complexes are also noted in the right precordial leads. Every second atrial beat is buried within the T-wave and produces a deformity of the T-wave in these leads. Whenever T-waves have a "deformed" or "pointy" (as in lead V1) appearance, one should consider the possibility of a buried P-wave as the cause.

54. **SB, rate 40.** Emergency physicians should be familiar with the common causes of drug-induced bradycardia: beta-receptor blocking medications, calcium channel blocking medications, digoxin, clonidine, opiates, and alcohols.

55. **SVT, rate 210.** The differential diagnosis of narrow-complex regular tachycardias includes ST, SVT, and atrial flutter. SVT is diagnosed based on the absence of P-waves or flutter-waves.

56. **Atrial fibrillation with rapid ventricular response and occasional PVCs, rate 140, RBBB, previous inferior and anterolateral MI.** The presence of a wide-complex irregular tachycardia should prompt consideration of atrial fibrillation with aberrant conduction (RBBB in this case), atrial fibrillation with WPW, and PVT. The presence of QRS complexes that maintain a constant morphology (with the exception of the PVCs) rules out the latter two diagnoses. Leftward axis is caused by a previous inferior MI.

57. **SR, rate 75, left atrial enlargement (LAE), non-specific T-wave flattening in inferior leads, U-waves in precordial leads suggestive of hypokalemia.** Left atrial enlargement is diagnosed when the P-wave is notched and has a duration >0·11 seconds in any of the leads; and when the downward terminal deflection of the P-wave in lead V1 has an amplitude ≥1 mm and duration ≥0·04 seconds. Prominent U-waves (suggestive of, though not pathognomonic for hypokalemia), are present in the precordial leads and produce a "camel hump"[2] effect next to the T-wave. When the T-waves and U-waves are fused, they produce the **appearance** of a prolonged QT-interval (although the **actual QT-interval** remains normal). Other ECG abnormalities associated with hypokalemia include PVCs and ventricular dysrhythmias, ST-segment depression, and decreased T-wave amplitude. This patient's serum potassium level was 2·9 mEq/L (normal 3·5–5·3 mEq/L).

58. **SR, rate 80, LAE, acute inferior MI, probable posterior MI (PMI).** Acute inferior MI is diagnosed based on the presence of ST-segment elevations in the inferior leads. ST-segment depression in the right precordial leads is often a reciprocal abnormality associated with acute inferior MI. However in this case, the presence of prominent R-waves in these leads is highly suggestive of posterior extension of the infarct. PMI was confirmed on echocardiography.

59. **SR, rate 80, recent inferior MI with persistent ischemia.** The presence of Q-waves in the inferior leads indicates transmural MI of uncertain age. However, there is slight ST-segment elevation and inverted T-waves indicating recent infarct with persistent ischemia.

60. **SR, rate 86, T-wave abnormality consistent with anteroseptal ischemia, prolonged QT-interval.** The differential diagnosis of prolonged QT-interval includes hypokalemia, hypomagnesemia, hypocalcemia, acute myocardial ischemia, elevated intracranial pressure, drugs with sodium channel blocking effects (for example cyclic antidepressants, quinidine, etc.), hypothermia, and congenital prolonged QT syndrome. Prolonged QT-interval due to myocardial ischemia is the initial consideration, given the T-inversions. However, the patient's baseline ECG (shown in case #51) demonstrated T-inversions as well. In this case, the prolonged QT-interval was due to hypomagnesemia; the serum magnesium level was 1·0 mEq/L (normal 1·4–2·0 mEq/L). The QT-interval normalized after IV replacement.

61. **SVT, rate 210.** The rhythm is a narrow-complex regular tachycardia. Retrograde P-waves are present immediately following the QRS complexes, common in SVT. ST-segment depression is present in the inferior and lateral leads. This is also a common abnormality in SVT and is of uncertain clinical significance. ST-segment depression in SVT is **not** a reliable indicator of ischemia and does not reproduce during exercise testing. The cause of ST-segment depression during SVT is uncertain.

62. **VT, rate 135.** The rhythm is a wide-complex regular tachycardia; the differential diagnosis includes ST with aberrant conduction, SVT with aberrant conduction, and VT. The absence of sinus activity rules out ST. The rhythm, therefore, should be assumed to be VT and treated as such. The presence of a rightward axis also strongly favors the diagnosis of VT. Electrophysiologic studies confirmed the diagnosis of VT.

63. **SR, rate 81, LAE, LVH with repolarization abnormality, acute pericarditis.** LVH often produces abnormalities in repolarization that cause ST-segment depression and asymmetric T-wave inversions in the lateral leads (I, aVL, V4–V6). LVH can also produce ST-segment elevation in the right precordial leads. Acute

pericarditis is diagnosed based on the presence of diffuse ST-segment elevation and PR-segment depression, most notable in the inferior and lateral leads.

64. **Atrial flutter with variable block, rate 130, previous septal MI, T-wave abnormality consistent with lateral ischemia.** Atrial flutter occurs in this case primarily with 2:1 AV conduction, but several areas of 3:1 AV conduction produce an irregular rhythm.

65. **SB, rate 40, LVH, T-wave abnormality consistent with anterolateral ischemia.** The T-wave inversions should not be assumed to be LVH-induced repolarization abnormalities for two reasons:
   - they are symmetric
   - they are present in more than just the lateral leads.

   SB in this case was induced by a heroin overdose. The patient was treated with naloxone, which resulted in a prompt increase in heart rate and resolution of the T-wave inversions. Common drug-induced causes of bradycardia in the emergency department setting include beta-receptor blocking medications, calcium channel blocking medications, digoxin, clonidine, opiates, and alcohols.

66. **SB, rate 56, WPW.** WPW is characterized by the triad of short PR-interval (<0·12 seconds), prolonged QRS-interval (>0·10 seconds), and slurring of the upstroke of the R-wave (delta-wave). Other causes of QRS-interval prolongation include hypothermia, hyperkalemia, aberrant intraventricular conduction (for example bundle branch block), ventricular ectopy, paced beats, and an extensive list of medications. WPW often simulates PMI and RBBB (or incomplete RBBB) by producing prominent R-waves in lead V1. Other causes of prominent R-waves in lead V1 include ventricular ectopy, RVH, acute right ventricular dilatation (right ventricular "strain," for example massive pulmonary embolism), hypertrophic cardiomyopathy, progressive muscular dystrophy, dextrocardia, and misplaced precordial electrodes. The prominent R-wave in lead V1 (defined as an R:S ratio >1) exists as a normal variant in only rare instances. See figure on p. 69.

67. **Atrial flutter with 2:1 AV conduction, rate 140.** The rhythm was initially misdiagnosed as SVT because of the absence of prominent flutter-waves in the inferior leads. However, whenever the ventricular rate in a narrow-complex tachycardia is 150 ± 20/minute, one should always scrutinize all 12 leads of the ECG to look for evidence of atrial flutter. In this case, definitive confirmation of atrial flutter is found in lead V1, which clearly shows atrial activity with a rate of 280/minute and 2:1 AV conduction. Lead V1 is often the best lead on the ECG to view the activity of the atrium.

68. **SR with first degree AV block, rate 66, LAE, non-specific intraventricular conduction delay and peaked T-waves suggestive of hyperkalemia.** The peaked T-waves associated with hyperkalemia tend to occur more frequently in the precordial leads. PR-interval and QRS-interval prolongation are markers of more severe levels of hyperkalemia. At even higher levels of hyperkalemia, high-grade AV blocks or ventricular dysrhythmias may occur. This patient's serum potassium level was 8·7 mEq/L (normal 3·5–5·3 mEq/L).

69. **SR with sinus arrhythmia, rate 60, acute anterior MI, inferior and lateral MI of uncertain age.** ST-segment elevation and prominent upright wide-based T-waves are present in the anterior leads, indicating acute anterior MI. The Q-waves in the inferior and lateral leads were the result of the patient's previous MI, but this was not known with certainty until a prior ECG was obtained. Prominent upright T-waves ("hyperacute T-waves") are often an early ECG marker of acute myocardial ischemia. Several other conditions as well, frequently produce prominent T-waves, including hyperkalemia, acute pericarditis, LVH, BER, bundle branch block, and pre-excitation syndromes. See figure on p. 70.

70. **SVT, rate 155, LVH.** Retrograde P-waves are seen following the QRS complexes, common with SVT. The leftward axis is accounted for by LVH.

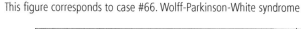

This figure corresponds to case #66. Wolff-Parkinson-White syndrome

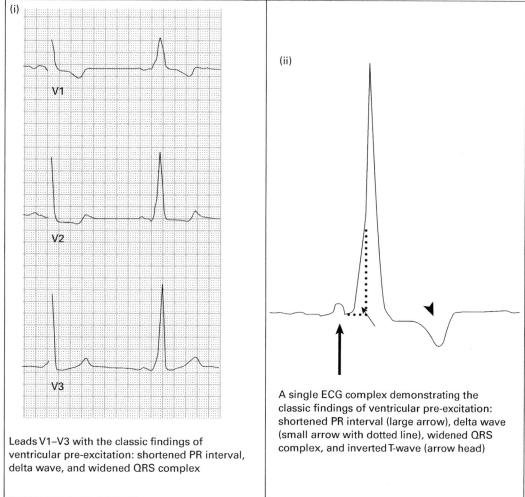

(i)

Leads V1–V3 with the classic findings of ventricular pre-excitation: shortened PR interval, delta wave, and widened QRS complex

(ii)

A single ECG complex demonstrating the classic findings of ventricular pre-excitation: shortened PR interval (large arrow), delta wave (small arrow with dotted line), widened QRS complex, and inverted T-wave (arrow head)

71. **SR with second degree AV block and 2:1 AV conduction, rate 40, LVH.** The atrial rate is 80/minute and regular. There are two P-waves for every one QRS complex; every other P-wave is non-conducted. When 2:1 conduction is present in second degree AV block, it is very difficult to distinguish with certainty between Mobitz I versus Mobitz II. Some helpful clues exist:
    - If Mobitz I is seen on another part of the ECG or rhythm strips, then Mobitz I is diagnosed.
    - If a bundle branch block or bifascicular block is present, it favors (although does not definitively prove) the diagnosis of Mobitz II.

    LVH is diagnosed here based on the presence of the R-wave amplitude in aVL >11 mm.

72. **ST, rate 105, acute anterior MI, LVH.** Q-waves have already developed in the anterior leads, indicating the presence of infarcted tissue. However, persistent ST-segment elevation indicates ongoing ischemia of myocardial tissue that has not yet infarcted.

73. **SR, rate 73, LAE, PRWP, T-wave abnormality consistent with lateral ischemia, non-specific T-wave flattening in inferior leads, low voltage.** The presence of PRWP (R-wave amplitude in lead V3 ≤3 mm) is suggestive of a previous anteroseptal MI, although in this case it was a normal variant. Low voltage is present, defined when the amplitudes of the QRS complexes in all of the limb leads is < 5 mm or when the amplitudes of the QRS complexes in all of the precordial

This figure corresponds to case #69. Prominent T-wave AMI

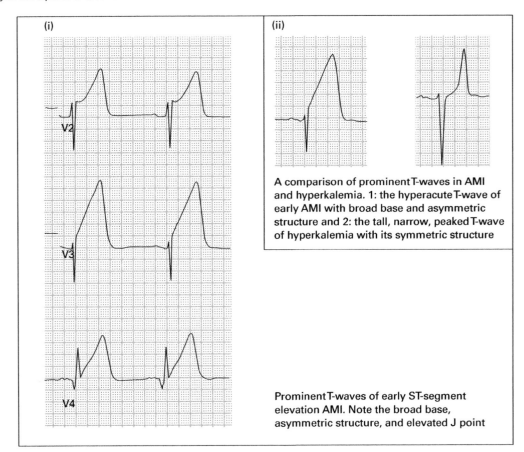

(i)

V2

V3

V4

(ii)

A comparison of prominent T-waves in AMI and hyperkalemia. 1: the hyperacute T-wave of early AMI with broad base and asymmetric structure and 2: the tall, narrow, peaked T-wave of hyperkalemia with its symmetric structure

Prominent T-waves of early ST-segment elevation AMI. Note the broad base, asymmetric structure, and elevated J point

leads is <10 mm. The differential diagnosis for low voltage includes myxedema, large pericardial effusion, large pleural effusion, end-stage cardiomyopathy, severe chronic obstructive pulmonary disease, severe obesity, infiltrative myocardial diseases, constrictive pericarditis, and prior massive MI. The patient in this case had severe emphysema.

74. **ST, rate 120, incomplete RBBB, T-wave abnormality consistent with inferior and anteroseptal ischemia.** This ECG contains all of the "classic" features of acute massive pulmonary embolism:
   - tachycardia
   - rightward axis
   - incomplete RBBB
   - S_I Q_{III} T_{III} (large S-wave in lead I, Q-wave in lead III, inverted T-wave in lead III)
   - simultaneous T-wave inversions in the inferior and anteroseptal leads.

Massive pulmonary embolism tends to cause acute right ventricular overload and dilatation (right ventricular "strain"), which often results in an incomplete or complete RBBB pattern. The Q-waves in leads III and aVF are not typical of MI-type of Q-waves, which are wider (>0·04 seconds duration). Simultaneous T-wave inversions in the inferior and anteroseptal leads should always prompt consideration of acute pulmonary embolism.[3] Acute pulmonary embolism should also strongly be considered in any patient with a rightward axis or a prominent R-wave in lead V1. This patient was admitted to the hospital for evaluation of her chest pain and dyspnea. Within an hour of her arrival on the telemetry unit, she suffered a cardiac arrest and died. Her autopsy revealed a large, lower extremity, deep venous thrombosis which had been producing a "shower" of pulmonary emboli (at least five noted at autopsy) over the preceding days.

75. **ST, rate 110, acute pericarditis.** Diffuse ST-segment elevations are present, prompting consideration of acute pericarditis, large MI, ventricular aneurysm, BER, and coronary vasospasm. PR-segment depressions, most prominently noted in the inferior leads, are highly specific for acute pericarditis. PR-segment elevation in lead aVR is often considered highly suggestive of acute pericarditis as well. However, this finding by itself should not exclude the other diagnoses; for example, PR-segment elevation in lead aVR is not an uncommon finding in acute MI. ST-segment depression in leads aVR and V1 is common in cases of acute pericarditis; however, the presence of ST-segment depression in any other leads is highly suggestive of acute MI ("reciprocal changes").

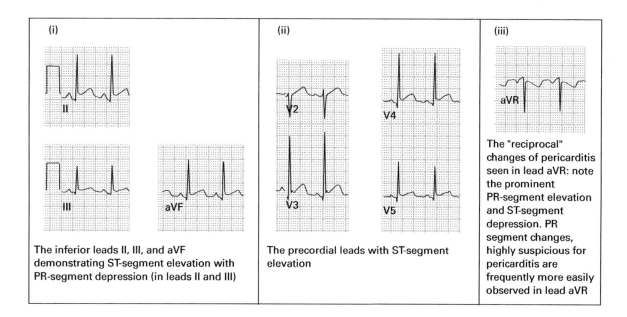

(i)	(ii)	(iii)
The inferior leads II, III, and aVF demonstrating ST-segment elevation with PR-segment depression (in leads II and III)	The precordial leads with ST-segment elevation	The "reciprocal" changes of pericarditis seen in lead aVR: note the prominent PR-segment elevation and ST-segment depression. PR segment changes, highly suspicious for pericarditis are frequently more easily observed in lead aVR

76. **SVT, rate 215.** ST-segment depression is present in the lateral leads and is of uncertain clinical significance in the presence of SVT.

77. **ST, rate 110, LAE, acute anterolateral MI.** The rightward axis is this case is caused by a lateral MI. Other causes of rightward axis include LPFB, RVH, acute (for example pulmonary embolism) and chronic (for example emphysema) lung disease, ventricular ectopy, hyperkalemia, and overdoses of sodium channel blocking drugs (for example cyclic antidepressants). Normal young or slender adults with a horizontally positioned heart can also demonstrate a rightward axis on the ECG. The patient demonstrates evidence of a large transmural MI (Q-waves) with ongoing ischemia (persistent ST-segment elevation).

78. **Atrial flutter with 2:1 AV conduction, rate 155.** The ventricular rate of 150 ± 20/minute should prompt consideration of atrial flutter and a search for flutter-waves. As with case #67, prominent flutter-waves are not seen in the inferior leads. However, lead V1 once again proves to be the lead where atrial activity is most clearly seen; small upright atrial beats at a rate of 310/minute are found. Leads I and aVL also provide a nice "view" of the atrial activity, although the flutter-waves here could easily be mistaken for artifact.

79. **VT, rate 155.** The QRS complexes are unusually wide (0·176 seconds), even in the setting of VT. The cause of this patient's tachydysrhythmia and wide-QRS complexes was hyperkalemia; his serum potassium level was 8·1 mEq/L (normal 3·5–5·3 mEq/L). The rhythm is approaching a sine-wave appearance due to the severity of abnormal ventricular conduction. The patient was initially treated for VT with lidocaine and amiodarone without improvement. He then developed asystole, after which intravenous calcium was administered ... but too late

to resuscitate the patient. Markedly wide QRS complexes, especially when bizarre in appearance, should always prompt early consideration of hyperkalemia.

80.   **Accelerated AV junctional rhythm, rate 70.** The rhythm is narrow-complex and regular without obvious P-waves preceding the QRS complexes. On the contrary, small P-waves are found following the QRS complexes (best seen in lead II and the mid-precordial leads), typical of an AV junctional rhythm. Because the rate is greater than the normal intrinsic AV junctional rate (40–60/minute), the rhythm is designated an **accelerated** AV junctional rhythm.

81.   **SR, rate 75, WPW.** The ECG demonstrates the classic triad of WPW:
    *   short PR-interval (<0·12 seconds)
    *   prolonged QRS-interval (>0·10 seconds), and
    *   slurring of the upstroke of the R-wave (delta-wave).

WPW can produce large Q-waves in the inferior leads, mimicking inferior MI. As demonstrated in case #66, WPW can also simulate posterior MI by producing large R-waves in lead V1. The leftward axis is caused by the abnormal conduction associated with WPW. Other causes of leftward axis include LAFB, LBBB, inferior myocardial infarction, left ventricular hypertrophy, ventricular ectopy, and paced beats.

82.   **ST with first degree AV block, rate 130, incomplete RBBB, T-wave abnormality consistent with inferior and anteroseptal ischemia.** The ECG is highly suggestive of acute massive pulmonary embolism (PE), much like case #74. Characteristic features of pulmonary embolism include:
    *   tachycardia
    *   rightward axis
    *   incomplete RBBB
    * $S_I Q_{III} T_{III}$ (large S-wave in lead I, Q-wave in lead III, inverted T-wave in lead III)
    *   simultaneous T-wave inversions in the inferior and anteroseptal leads.

Acute right heart "strain" from pulmonary embolism often results in an enlarged "pointy" P-wave in lead V1, as seen in this case. This patient did prove to have pulmonary emboli causing his symptoms.

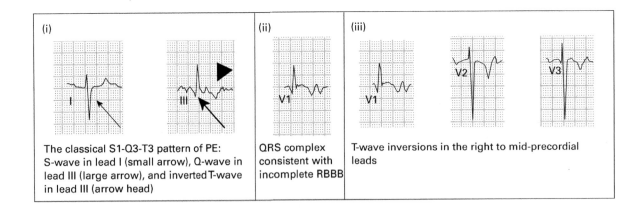

(i)

The classical S1-Q3-T3 pattern of PE: S-wave in lead I (small arrow), Q-wave in lead III (large arrow), and inverted T-wave in lead III (arrow head)

(ii)

QRS complex consistent with incomplete RBBB

(iii)

T-wave inversions in the right to mid-precordial leads

83.   **SR with first degree AV block, rate 70, previous inferior MI.** This ECG demonstrates a marked first degree AV block (0·445 seconds) due to severe AV nodal disease. When patients have marked first degree AV blocks, the P-waves can sometimes be mistaken for U-waves (for example in leads V3–V6). Close attention to all 12 leads helps clarify P-waves versus U-waves.

84. **Atrial flutter with variable block and occasional PVCs, rate 110, previous inferior MI.** The rhythm is narrow-complex and irregular, prompting consideration of atrial flutter with variable block, atrial fibrillation, and MAT. Prominent flutter-waves are found in the inferior leads, clarifying the diagnosis.

85. **SB with first degree AV block, rate 42, acute inferior MI.** Bradycardia, first degree AV block, and second degree AV block type I (Mobitz I) are all common complications of acute inferior MI. These are usually vagally-mediated and respond well to atropine, as did this patient's rhythm. Reciprocal ST-segment depression is present in leads I, aVL, and the anteroseptal leads, typical of inferior MIs.

86. **SR, rate 92, LAE, right atrial enlargement (RAE), acute inferior and posterior MI (PMI).** LAE is diagnosed based on the presence of P-wave duration ≥0·12 seconds and a downward terminal deflection of the P-wave in lead V1 that has a negative amplitude ≥1 mm and a duration of ≥0·04 seconds. RAE is diagnosed based on the P-wave amplitude in any of the inferior leads >2·5 mm. Posterior extension of the inferior MI is indicated by the presence of ST-segment depression, upright T-waves, and tall R-waves in the right precordial leads. The prominent ST-segment depression and T-wave inversions in the lateral leads may represent reciprocal changes from the acute inferior MI or lateral subendocardial injury. Subsequent echocardiography and coronary angiography confirmed PMI but no evidence of lateral injury in this patient.

87. **SR, rate 66, LAFB, acute anterolateral MI.** LAFB is diagnosed based on the presence of LAD, an rS complex (small R-wave and large S-wave) in lead III, and qR complexes (small Q-waves and large R-waves) in leads I and aVL. ST-segment elevation is present throughout the precordial leads and in leads I and aVL, consistent with an acute large anterior and lateral MI. Slight reciprocal ST-segment depression is present in leads III and aVF.

88. **SB with first degree AV block, rate 55, PRWP, low voltage.** PRWP, defined when the R-wave amplitude in lead V3 ≤3 mm, has many causes. It may be caused by a prior anteroseptal MI, LVH, by abnormally high placement of the mid-precordial electrodes, or may simply be a normal variant. This ECG also exhibits low voltage. Low voltage is diagnosed when the amplitudes of the QRS complexes in all of the limb leads are ≤5 mm or when the amplitudes of the QRS complexes in all of the precordial leads are ≤10 mm. The differential diagnosis of low voltage includes myxedema, large pericardial effusion, large pleural effusion, end-stage cardiomyopathy, severe chronic obstructive pulmonary disease, severe obesity, infiltrative myocardial diseases, constrictive pericarditis, and prior massive MI. Low voltage in this case was attributed to the patient's obesity.

89. **SR with PVCs leading to polymorphic ventricular tachycardia (PVT), torsade de pointes (TDP).** The first and third QRS complexes on the ECG appear to be sinus beats conducted to the ventricle (there is a P-wave preceding the third QRS; presumably, therefore, a P-wave precedes the first QRS as well but is cut-off by the ECG). These QRS complexes are wide, indicating aberrant conduction of some type. The second QRS complex is a PVC. Following the third QRS complex, a PVC occurs during the final portion of the T-wave (R-on-T phenomenon), inducing PVT. The ensuing rhythm is wide-complex and irregular. The differential diagnosis for wide-complex irregular rhythms includes PVT, atrial fibrillation with WPW, and atrial fibrillation with aberrant conduction (for example bundle branch block). Atrial fibrillation with aberrant conduction is ruled out based on the presence of QRS complexes that vary significantly in morphology and amplitude. Atrial fibrillation with WPW is ruled out because there is no evidence during the first portion of the ECG of WPW (SR with short PR-interval or delta-wave). Atrial fibrillation with WPW also tends to be less chaotic than what is found here. TDP is a type of PVT that occurs in the presence of a prolonged QT-interval. It has a characteristic appearance in that the polarity and amplitude of the QRS complexes appear to rotate around a central axis. This patient was severely hypomagnesemic and hypokalemic. His baseline rhythm strips demonstrated a prolonged QT-interval due to the electrolyte abnormalities, predisposing him to this tachydysrhythmia. He was successfully defibrillated and he did well.

90. **SVT, rate 210.** The rhythm is narrow-complex and regular; the differential includes ST, SVT, and atrial flutter. Close inspection for atrial activity reveals retrograde P-waves, often present in SVT, best noted in lead V1. Electrical alternans and mild ST-segment depressions are noted in some leads. These abnormalities are also occasionally found in SVT and are without clinical significance.

91. **ST, rate 120, incomplete RBBB, T-wave abnormality consistent with inferior and anteroseptal ischemia.** The ECG is highly suggestive of acute massive pulmonary embolism, similar to cases #74 and #82. The ECG abnormalities of pulmonary embolism are transient in nature, usually lasting weeks to months. However, RVH and its associated ECG abnormalities may develop if chronic pulmonary hypertension develops. A ventilation-perfusion scan in this patient demonstrated multiple pulmonary emboli.

92. **SR, rate 85, incomplete RBBB, T-wave abnormality consistent with inferior and anterolateral ischemia.** In 1982, Wellens and colleagues[1] described two T-wave morphologies in the mid-precordial leads that are highly specific for a large proximal left anterior descending artery (LAD) obstructing lesion. The more common morphology is a symmetric and deeply inverted T-wave appearance, as shown in this case. The less common type is the biphasic T-wave morphology, as shown in case #33. The T-wave abnormality, which has come to be known as Wellens' sign, usually persists even in the pain-free state. Medical treatment is often unsuccessful in preventing MI or death; invasive therapy with angioplasty or stent placement is most successful. This patient was found to have a >90% proximal LAD obstructing lesion. She was successfully treated with angioplasty.

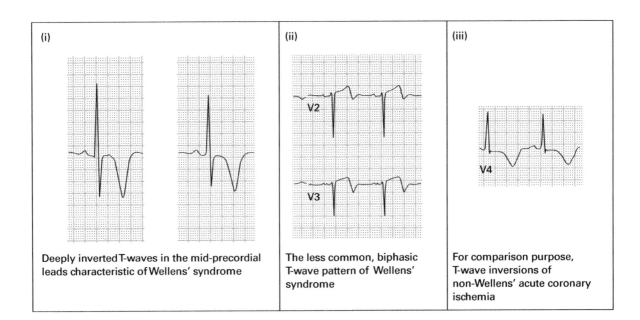

(i) Deeply inverted T-waves in the mid-precordial leads characteristic of Wellens' syndrome

(ii) The less common, biphasic T-wave pattern of Wellens' syndrome

(iii) For comparison purpose, T-wave inversions of non-Wellens' acute coronary ischemia

93. **SR, rate 88, persistent juvenile T-wave pattern.** Normal young adults, especially women, may have a persistence of the T-wave inversions in leads V1–V3 that are usually present in children and adolescents. This is referred to as a "persistent juvenile T-wave pattern." These T-wave inversions are asymmetric and shallow. If the inversions are symmetric or deep, myocardial ischemia should be assumed.

94. **ST, rate 140, LVH.** ST or atrial fibrillation with rapid ventricular response is common in severe hyperthyroidism. These tachydysrhythmias may precede other clinical manifestations of disease. Hyperthyroidism was confirmed in this patient.

95. **SR with first degree AV block, LBBB.** LBBB is associated with characteristic repolarization abnormalities that all emergency physicians should know well. ST-segments are displaced in an opposite direction to the QRS complex ("discordant" with the QRS complex). ST-segments that are deflected in the same direction as ("concordant" with) the QRS complex may indicate acute MI or ischemia. Various authors have proposed criteria that indicate when acute MI or ischemia should be considered in the presence of LBBB. Although none of these criteria have been shown to be 100% accurate, emergency physicians should be familiar with the most well-known of these criteria, proposed by Sgarbossa[4] in 1996. She stated that acute MI should be considered in the presence of LBBB when:
    - ST-segment elevation of ≥1 mm is concordant with the QRS complex
    - ST-segment depression of ≥1 mm is present in leads V1, V2, or V3
    - ST-segment elevation of ≥5 mm is discordant with the QRS complex.

96. **SR with first degree AV block, rate 80, acute inferior, lateral, and right ventricular (RV) MI.** ST-segment elevation consistent with acute MI is present in the inferior and lateral leads. Reciprocal ST-segment depression is present in leads I and aVL. Acute inferior MI is usually associated with reciprocal ST-segment depression in the right precordial leads as well. However, when ST-segment depression is limited to lead V2 and the ST-segment in lead V1 is either elevated or isoelectric, RV MI is suggested. ST-segment elevation in lead III that exceeds the ST-segment elevation in lead II is also suggestive of RV MI.

97. **Right-sided precordial leads (same patient as in case #96): SR with first degree AV block, rate 90, acute inferior and RV MI.** Right-sided precordial leads are placed across the right side of the chest to evaluate for RV extension of acute inferior or lateral MI. Any ST-segment elevation in the (right) lateral precordial leads indicates acute RV MI.

98. **SR, rate 75, LAE, prolonged QT, acute anterolateral MI.** Q-waves have already developed in the anterior and lateral leads, but there is some persistent ST-segment elevation in leads V1–V2 as well as inverted T-waves diffusely, suggesting the presence of persistent ischemia. The slightly prolonged QT-interval in this case was due to myocardial ischemia. Other causes of prolonged QT-interval include hypokalemia (actually due to fusion of T-waves and U-waves), hypomagnesemia, hypocalcemia, elevated intracranial pressure, drugs with sodium channel blocking effects (for example cyclic antidepressants, quinidine, etc.), and congenital prolonged QT syndrome.

99. **Ectopic atrial rhythm, rate 60, BER.** P-waves originating from the sinus node are upright in leads I, II, III, and aVF. The presence of inverted P-waves in any of these leads suggests an ectopic origin, either atrial or AV junctional. The PR-interval is ≥0·12 seconds, consistent with an atrial origin of the P-waves. AV junctional rhythms can sometimes produce inverted P-waves preceding the QRS complex, but the PR-interval will be <0·12 seconds. Diffuse ST-segment elevation is present, in this case due to BER. Clues that suggest BER include the patient's young age; the presence of concave upwards ST-segment elevation; the absence of reciprocal ST-segment depression, inverted T-waves, and Q-waves; and the absence of PR-segment depression. The ST-segment elevation in BER is usually most prominent in anterolateral precordial leads.

100. **SR, rate 95, peaked T-waves consistent with hyperkalemia.** The T-waves are only slightly peaked and the QRS-interval is narrow. This might suggest mild hyperkalemia; however, this patient's serum potassium level was 8·2 mEq/L (normal 3·5–5·3 mEq/L). Contrast the "mild" ECG abnormalities in this case with the pre-cardiac arrest ECG in case #79, in which the patient's serum potassium level was 8·1 mEq/L. Although the ECG is fairly sensitive at detecting hyperkalemia, there is a poor correlation between ECG abnormalities and specific serum potassium levels.

References

1. de Zwann C, Bar FW, Wellens HJJ. Characteristic electrocardiographic pattern indicating a critical stenosis high in left anterior descending coronary artery in patients admitted because of impending myocardial infarction. *Am Heart J* 1982;**103**:730–6.
2. Marriott HJL. *Marriott's Manual of Electrocardiography*. Orlando, FL: Trinity Press, 1995, p. 141.
3. Marriott HJL. *Pearls & Pitfalls in Electrocardiography*, *2nd edn*. Baltimore, MD: Williams & Wilkins, 1998, p. 134.
4. Sgarbossa EB, Pinski SL, Barbagelata A *et al*. Electrocardiographic diagnosis of evolving acute myocardial infarction in the presence of left bundle-branch block, GUSTO-1 (Global Utilization of Streptokinase and Tissue Plasminogen Activator for Occluded Coronary Arteries) Investigators. *N Engl J Med* 1996;**334**:481–7.

Part 2

Case histories

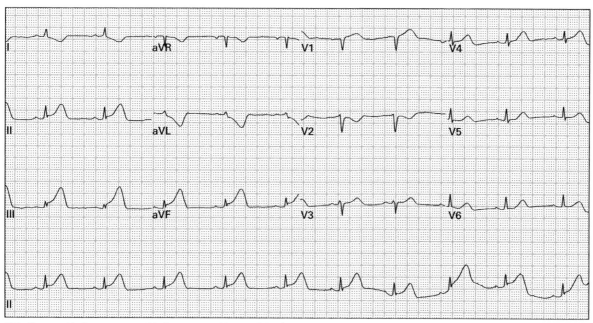

101. 43 year old obese woman with dyspnea, vomiting, and diaphoresis

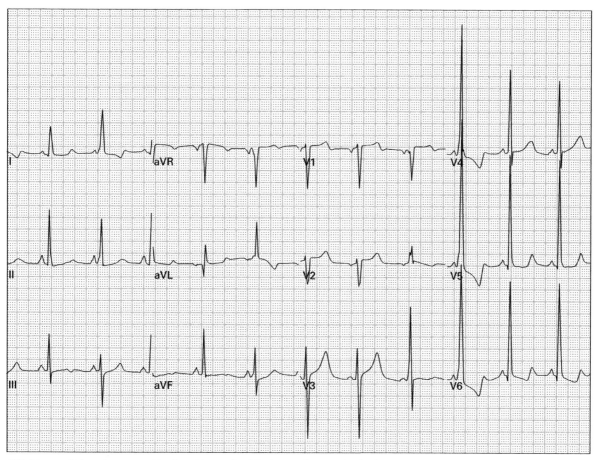

102. 54 year old homeless man with a long history of palpitations and syncopal episodes

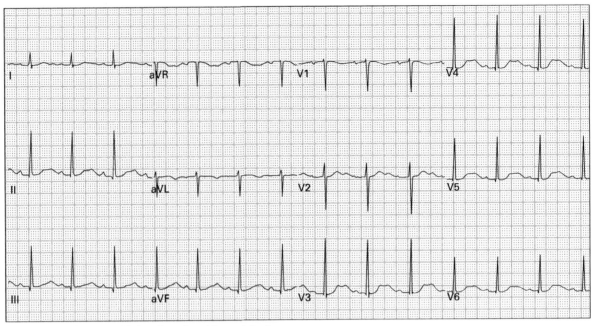

103. 46 year old woman with four days of vomiting and diarrhea

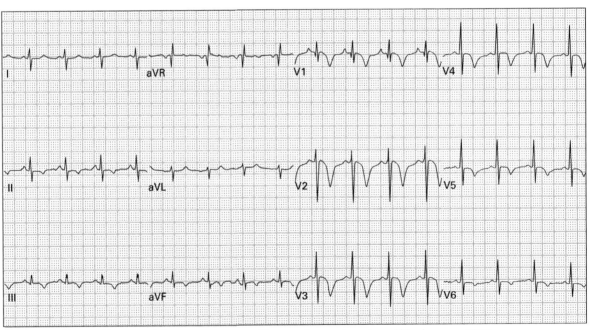

104. 58 year old man with metastatic lung cancer presents with severe dyspnea, hypoxia, and blood pressure 88/45

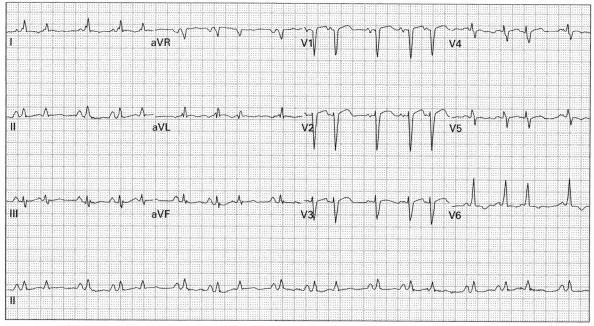

105. 70 year old woman with vomiting and diarrhea

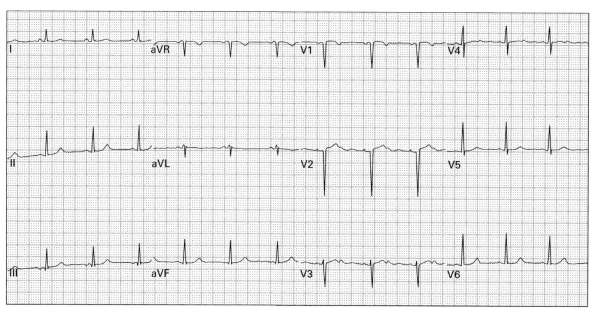

106. 64 year old woman presents after a syncopal episode

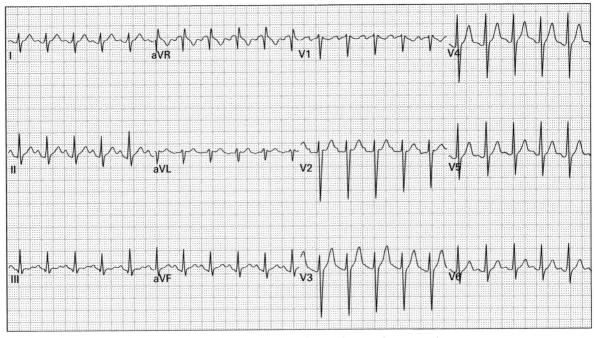

107. 29 year old man presents with altered mentation and agitated behavior after an unknown overdose

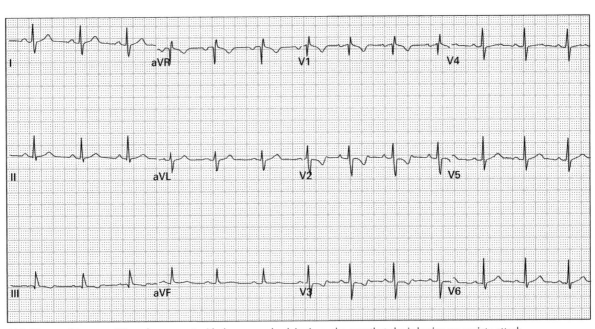

108. 18 year old woman 26 weeks pregnant with dyspnea and palpitations; she says that she is having an anxiety attack

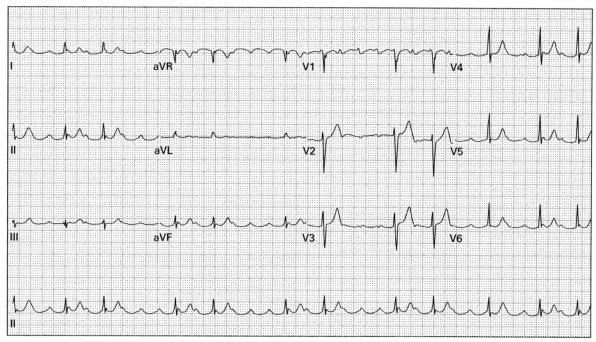

109. 48 year old man with history of congestive heart failure presents with nausea, vomiting, and weakness

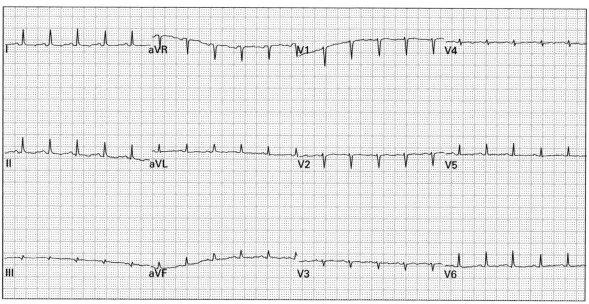

110. 40 year old woman with dyspnea and chest ache; blood pressure is 85/50

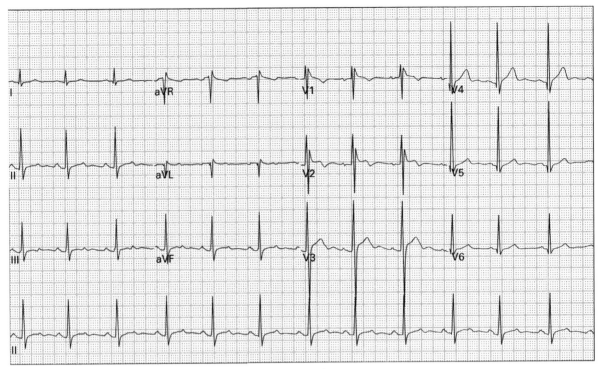

111. 37 year old man presents after a syncopal episode, now asymptomatic

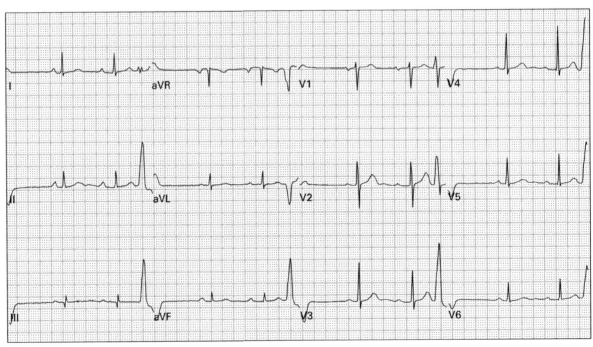

112. 53 year old woman with lightheadedness

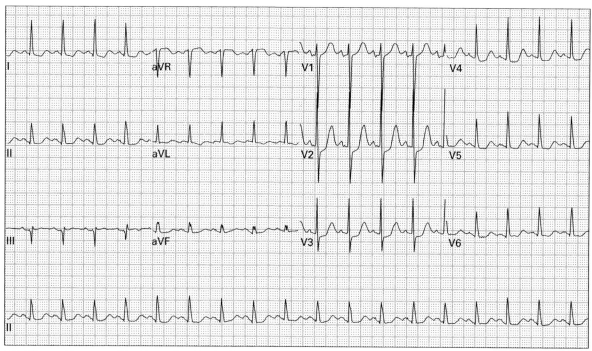

113. 75 year old woman with midsternal and back ache

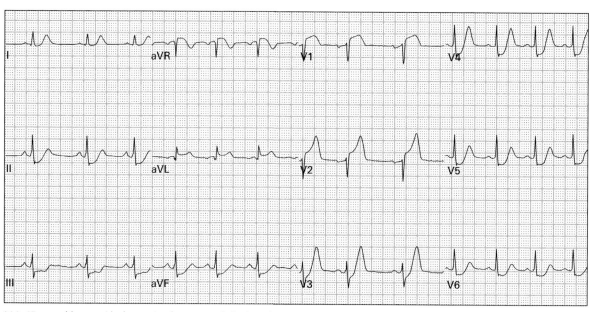

114. 45 year old man with chest pain, dyspnea, and diaphoresis

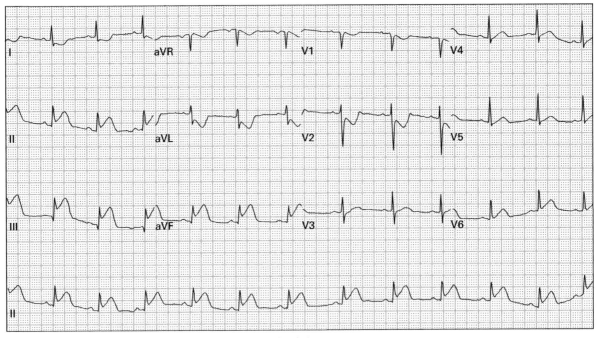

115. 44 year old woman with chest pressure, vomiting, and lightheadedness

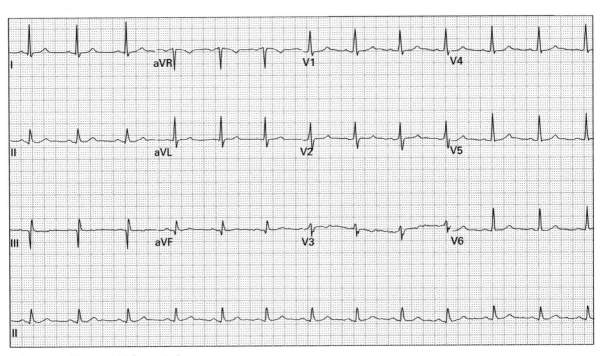

116. 54 year old man with left arm tingling

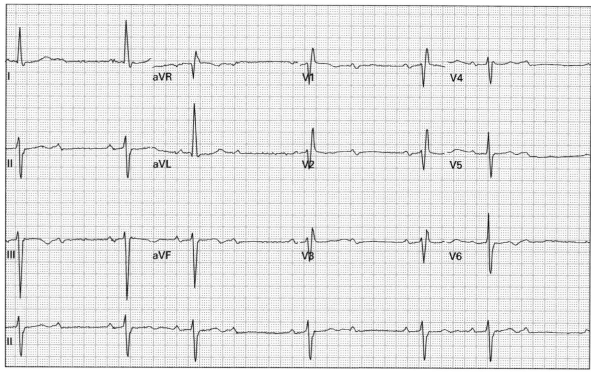

117. 83 year old woman with severe lightheadedness and nausea

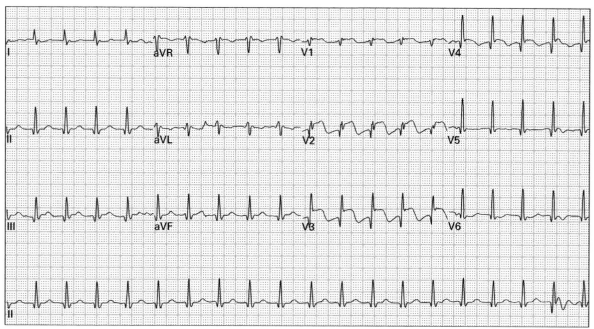

118. 48 year old man with chest pain and palpitations

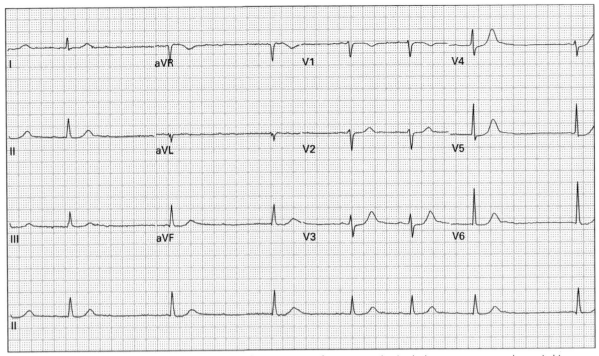

119. 67 year old man with a history of chronic atrial fibrillation presents after a syncopal episode; he reports a recent change in his medications

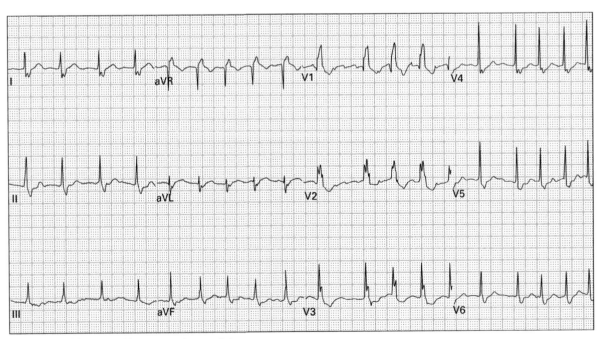

120. 74 year old woman with nausea and severe fatigue

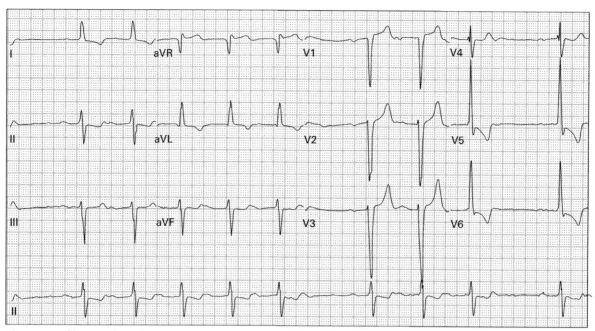

121. 71 year old man with weakness and nausea

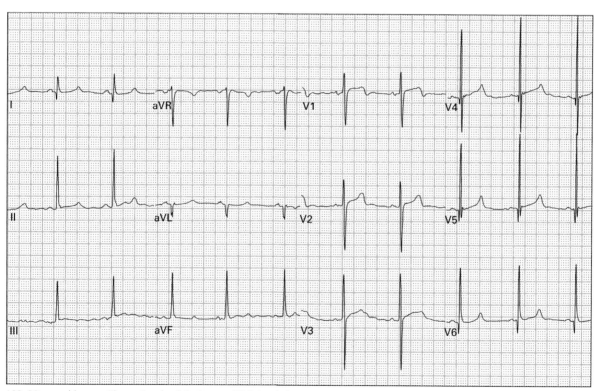

122. 30 year old man with exertional palpitations and lightheadedness

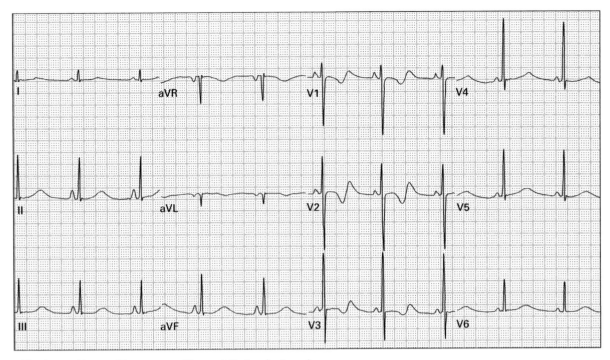

123. 49 year old man with nausea, vomiting, and diarrhea for three days

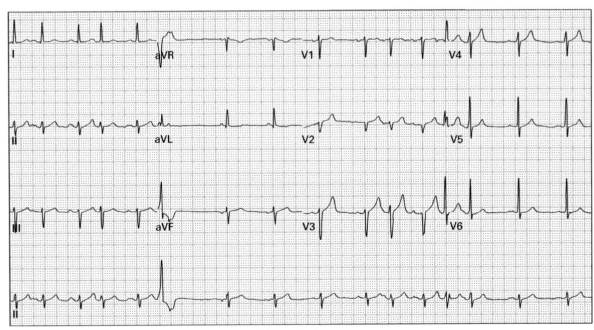

124. 72 year old man with severe emphysema presents with increasing dyspnea

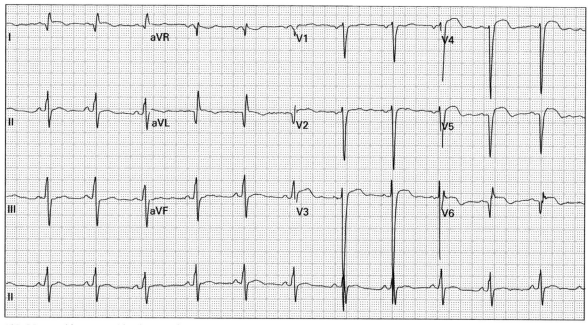

125. 56 year old woman with a history of a prior MI gets a pre-admission ECG; she is being admitted for cellulitis of the leg; she has no cardiopulmonary symptoms

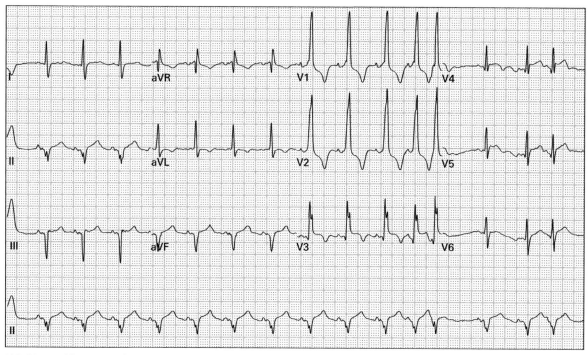

126. 87 year old woman with vomiting and dyspnea

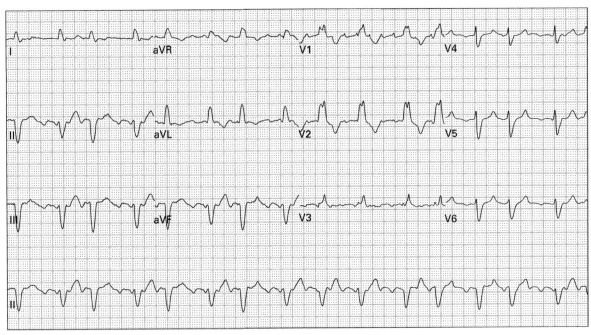

127. 66 year old woman with lightheadedness

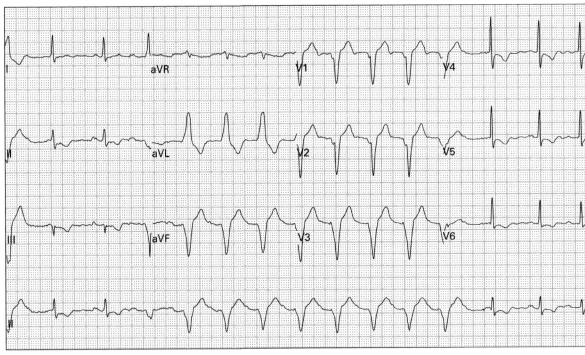

128. 54 year old man with chest pain and intermittent palpitations

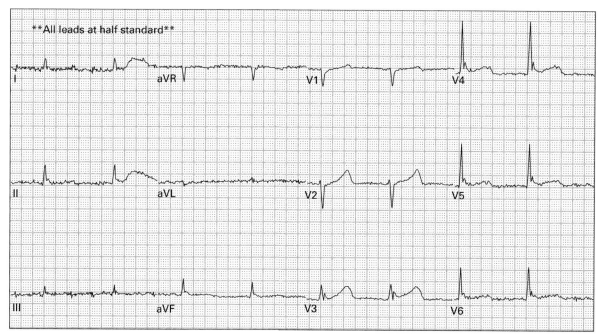

129. 53 year old alcoholic man with decreased level of consciousness

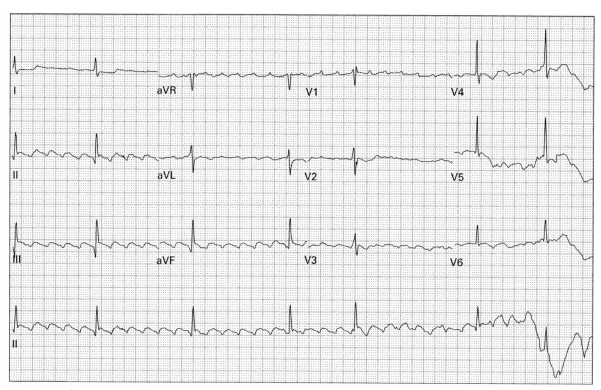

130. 67 year old woman with history of congestive heart failure presents with exertional lightheadedness, nausea, and vomiting

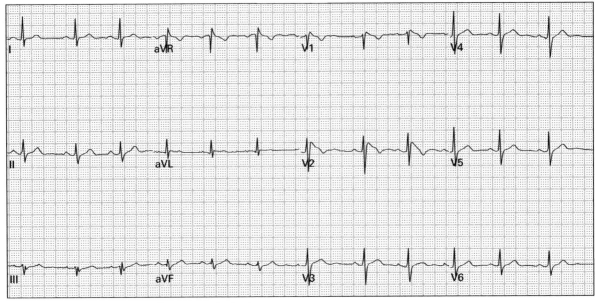

131. 30 year old woman presents after a syncopal episode

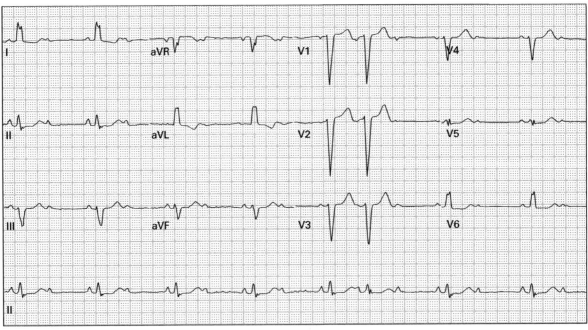

132. 58 year old woman with chest pain and weakness

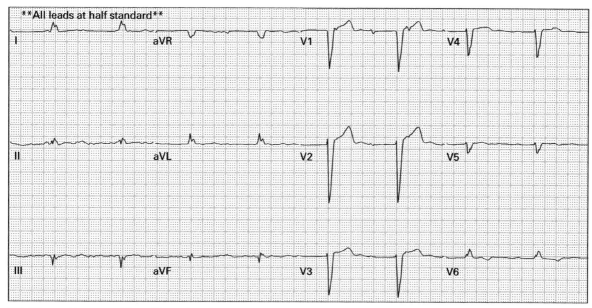

133. 74 year old woman with vomiting and weakness

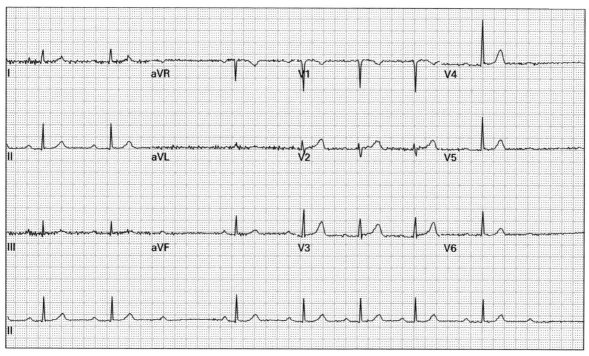

134. 41 year old woman with exertional lightheadedness

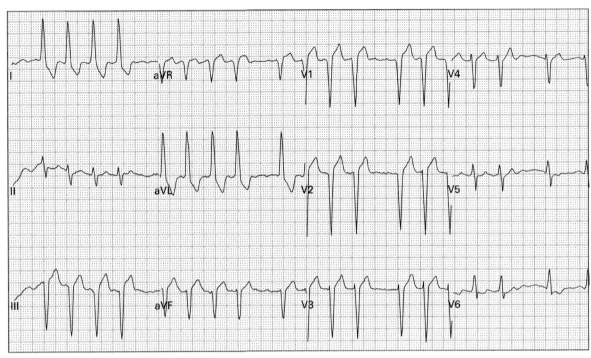

135. 91 year old woman with lightheadedness and dyspnea

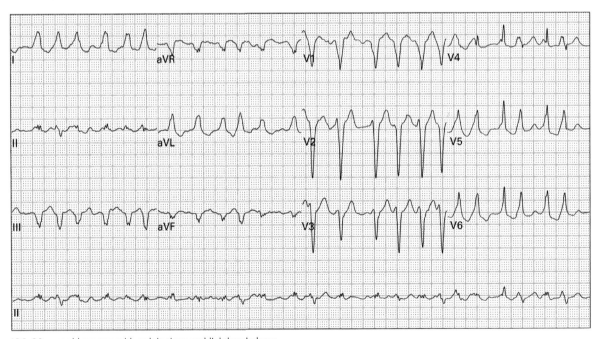

136. 30 year old woman with palpitations and lightheadedness

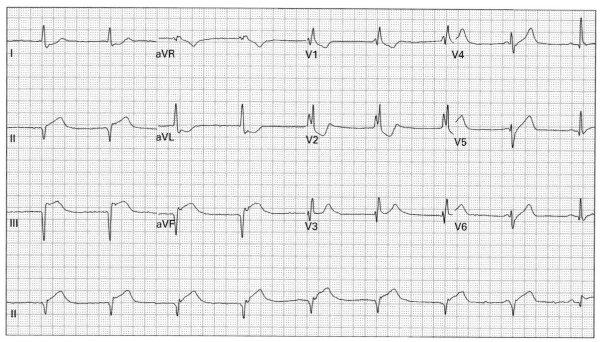

137. 86 year old man with chest pain radiating to both arms

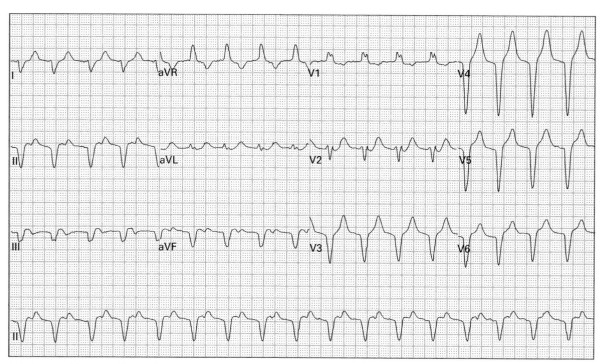

138. 86 year old man two hours after receiving intravenous streptokinase for acute MI; asymptomatic, blood pressure 125/70

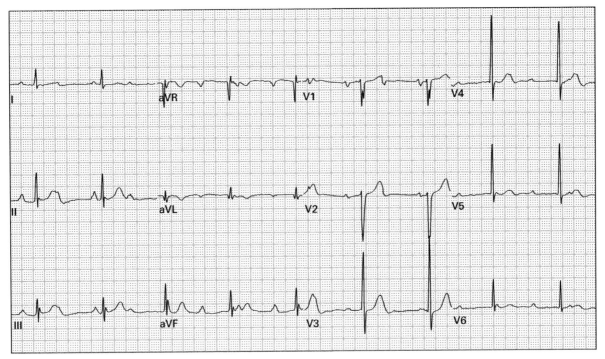

139. 54 year old man with lightheadedness during walking

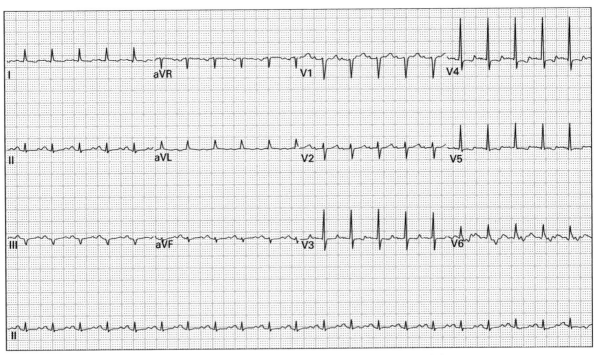

140. 39 year old man with severe alcoholic cardiomyopathy presents with palpitations and lightheadedness

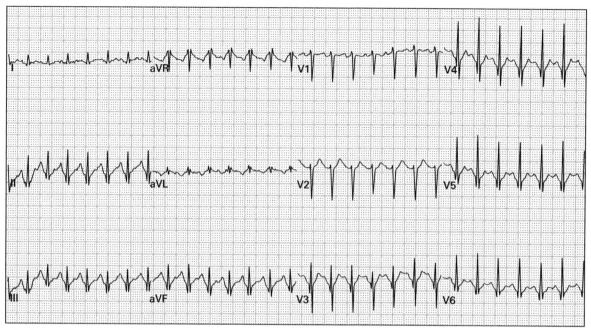

141. 43 year old woman with high fever, productive cough, and vomiting for one week

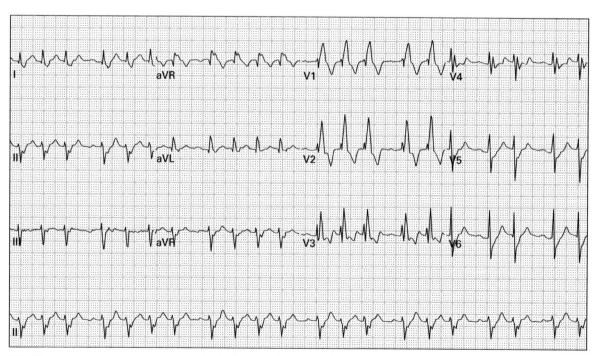

142. 47 year old man presents after a syncopal episode; now only reports palpitations

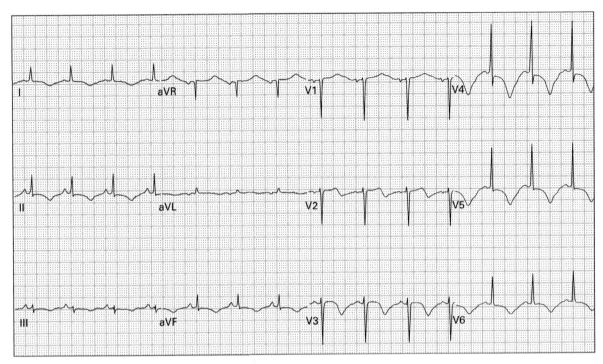

143. 62 year old woman presents unconscious

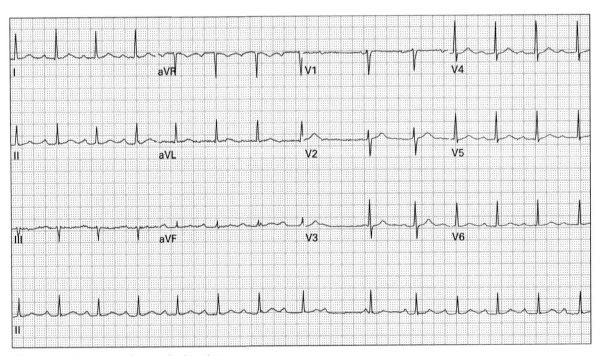

144. 63 year old woman with generalized weakness

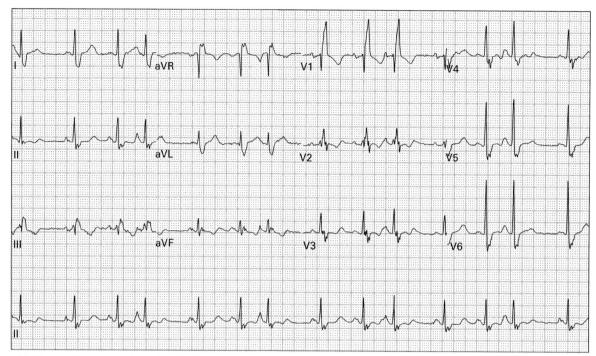

145. 73 year old woman with cough and wheezing

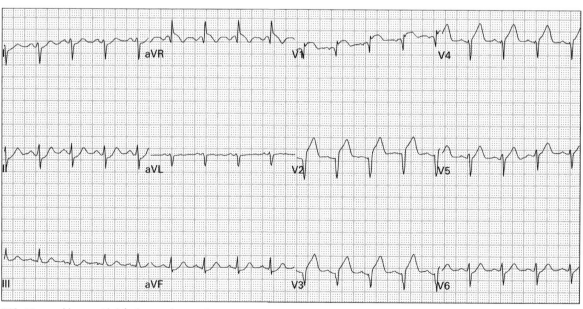

146. 44 year old man with left chest and arm pain

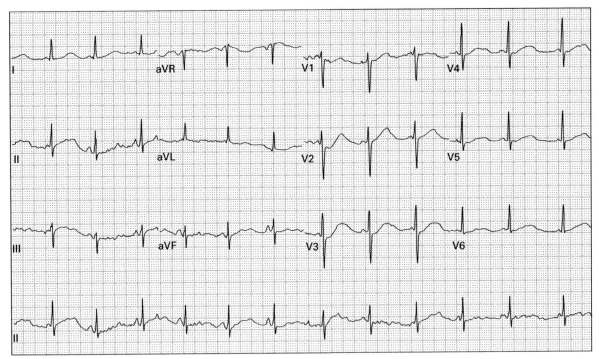

147. 57 year old man with history of schizophrenia presents after an overdose

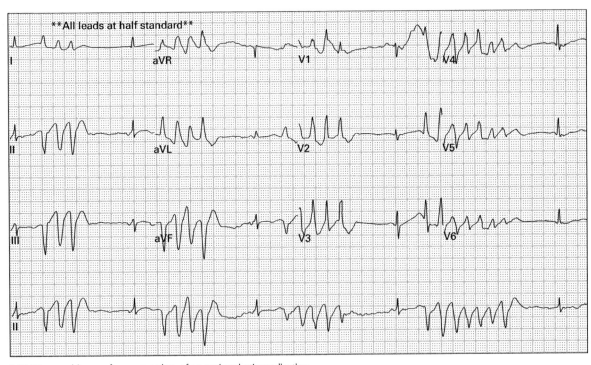

148. 57 year old man after an overdose of an antipsychotic medication

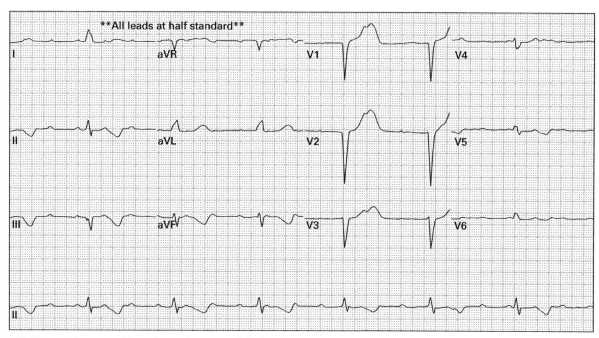

149. 68 year old woman with weakness, dyspnea, and diaphoresis

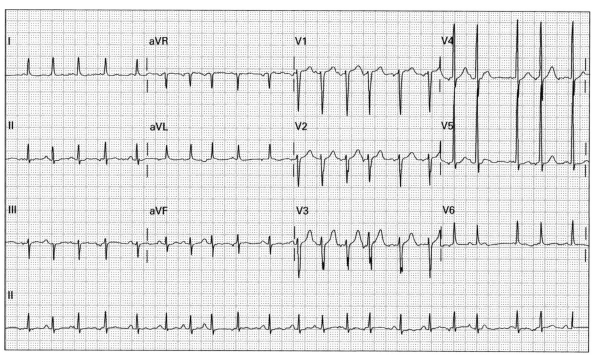

150. 65 year old man with history of emphysema presents with cough and fever

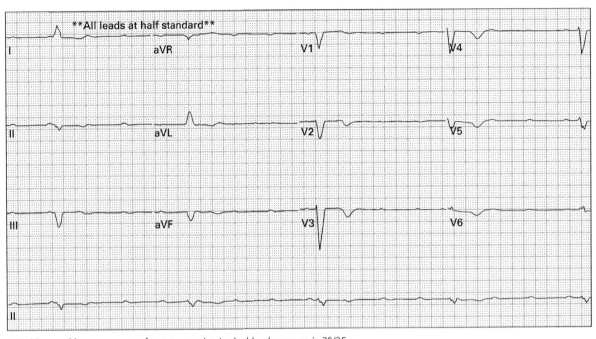

151. 82 year old man presents after a syncopal episode; blood pressure is 70/35

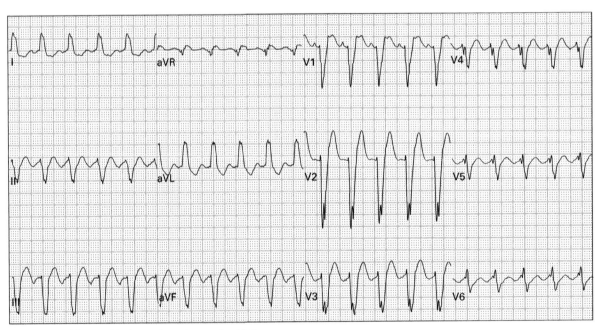

152. 67 year old man with chest ache and generalized fatigue

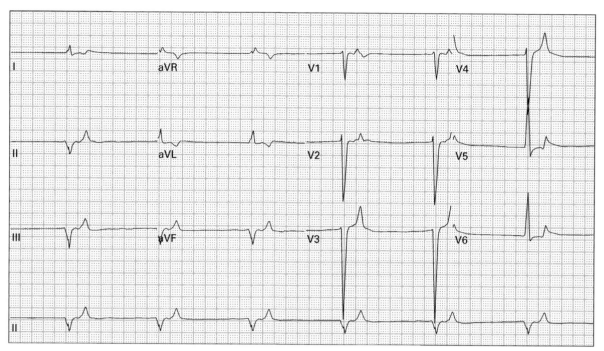

153. 44 year old man with chronic kidney disease presents with weakness and nausea

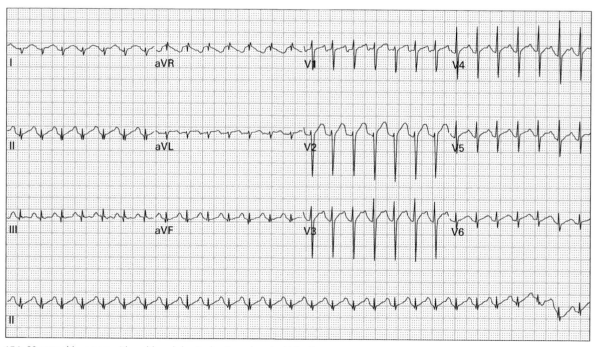

154. 23 year old woman with sudden abdominal pain and vaginal bleeding

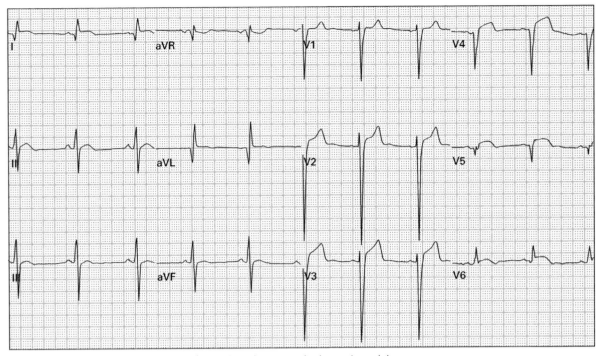

155. 44 year old woman with prior history of MI with productive cough, chest pain, and dyspnea

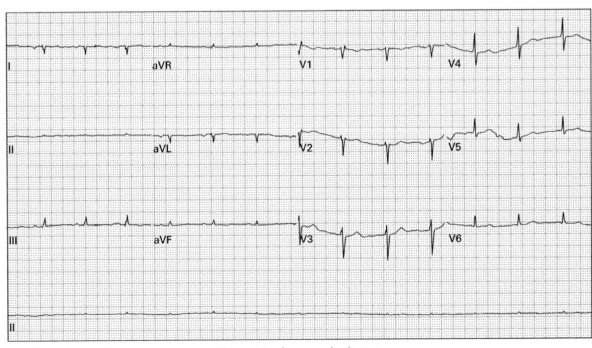

156. 52 year old man with lung cancer presents with worsening dyspnea and orthopnea

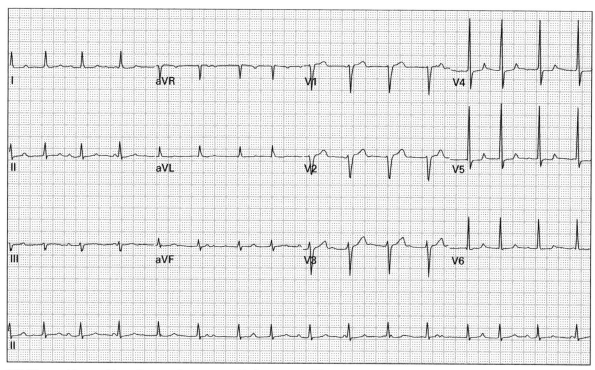

157. 39 year old man with cardiomyopathy presents with dyspnea on mild exertion

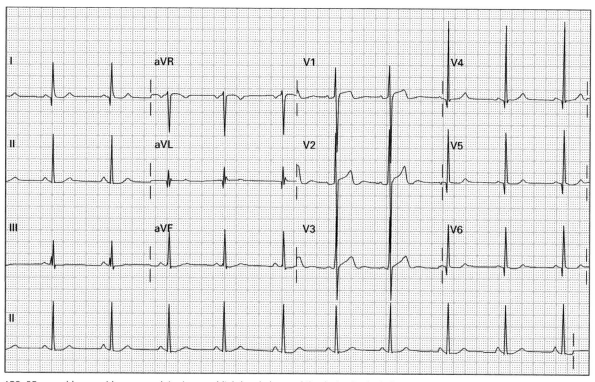

158. 25 year old man with severe palpitations and lightheadedness while playing basketball

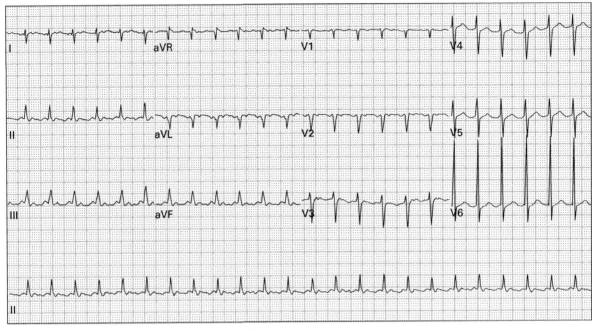

159. 53 year old alcoholic man with vomiting and palpitations

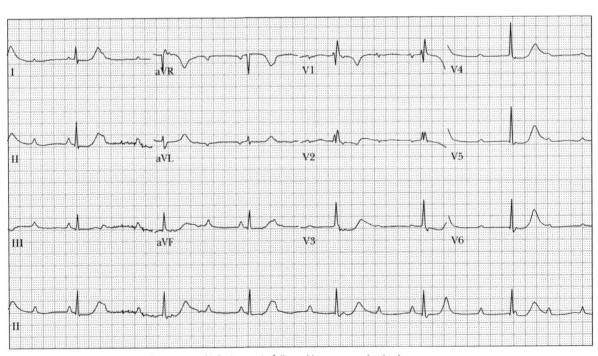

160. 51 year old woman reports three hours of left chest pain followed by a syncopal episode

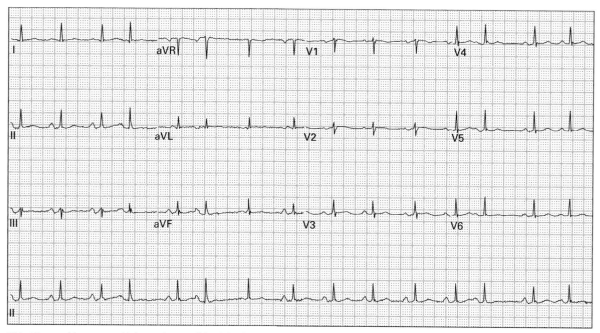

161. 49 year old woman with intermittent mild palpitations

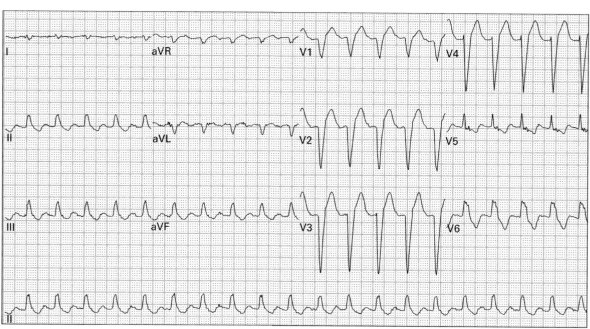

162. 61 year old man with fever, productive cough, and dyspnea

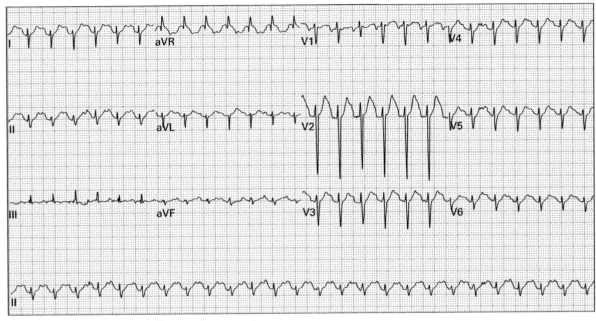

163. 37 year old woman presents after an unknown overdose

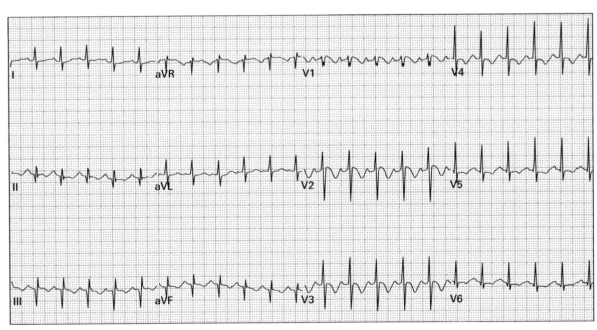

164. 50 year old man with chest pressure and dyspnea

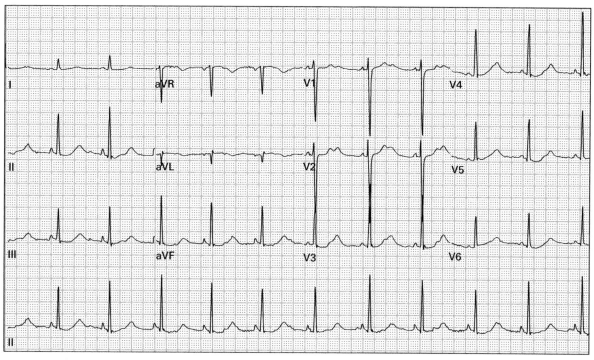

165. 31 year old woman with bulimia presents with severe weakness

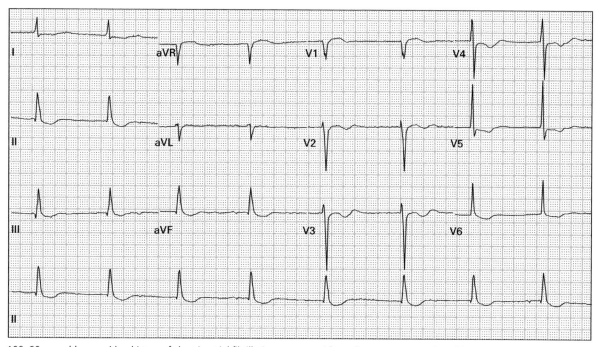

166. 66 year old man with a history of chronic atrial fibrillation presents with weakness, nausea, and vomiting

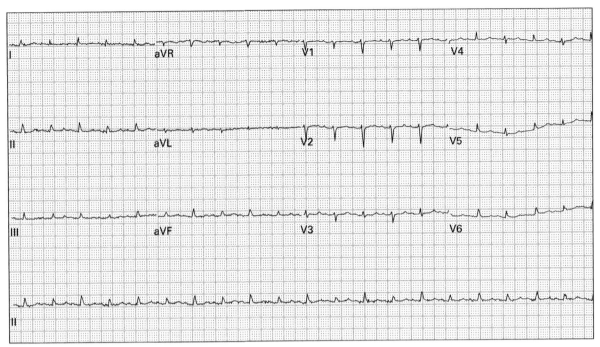

167. 54 year old woman with metastatic breast cancer presents with shortness of breath; blood pressure is 85/45

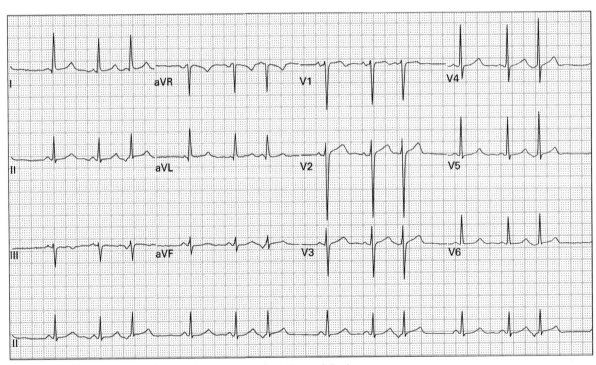

168. 53 year old man presents with palpitations, two days of vomiting and diarrhea

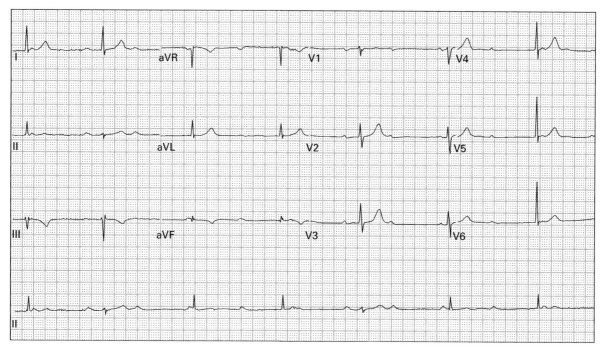

169. 54 year old man with severe lightheadedness and nausea

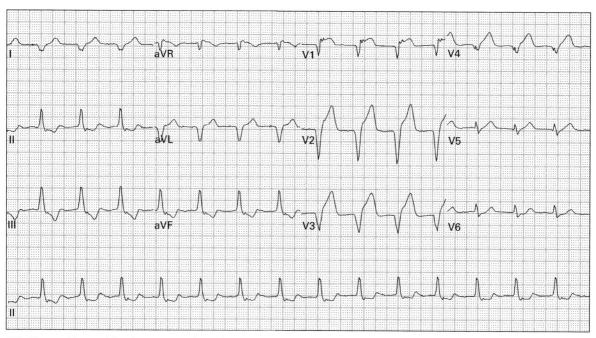

170. 78 year old man with palpitations one hour after receiving intravenous thrombolytics for an acute MI; blood pressure is 140/85

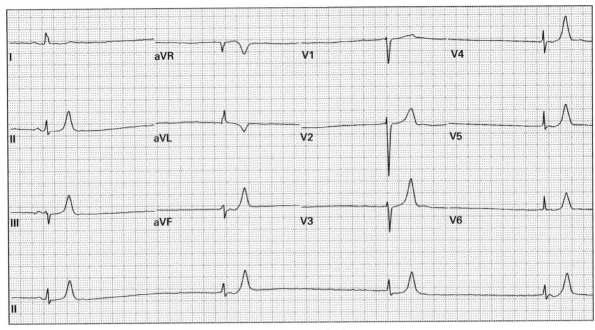

171. 60 year old woman with one week of fevers, anorexia, vomiting, and diarrhea

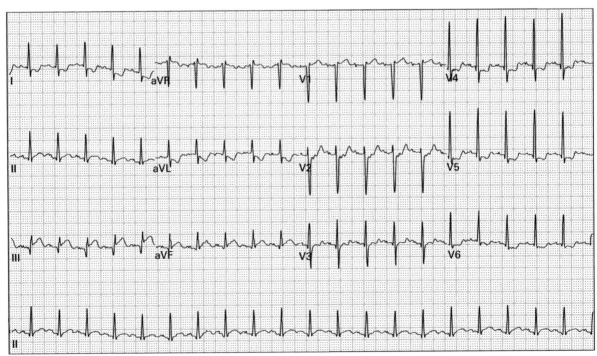

172. 75 year old man with dyspnea and nausea

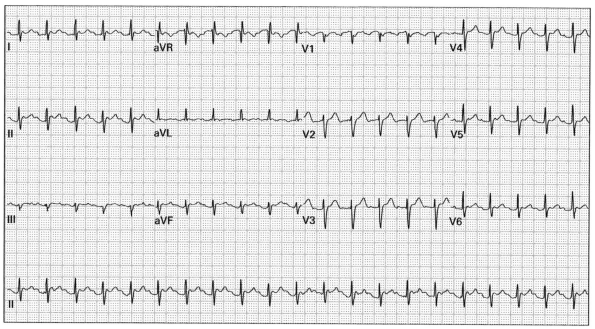

173. 52 year old man with chest pain and palpitations

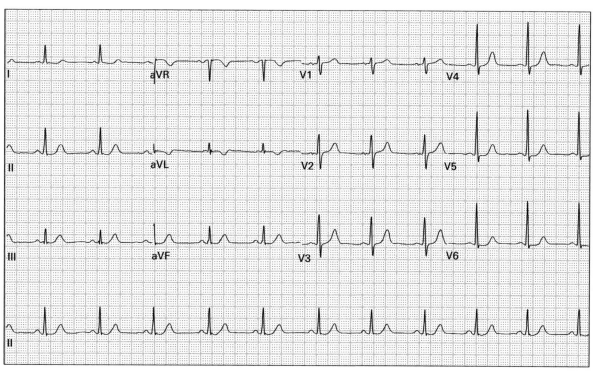

174. 56 year old man with chest pain, diaphoresis, and vomiting

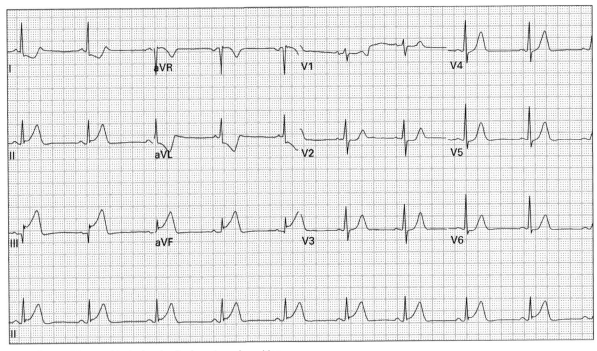

175. 56 year old man with chest pain, diaphoresis, and vomiting

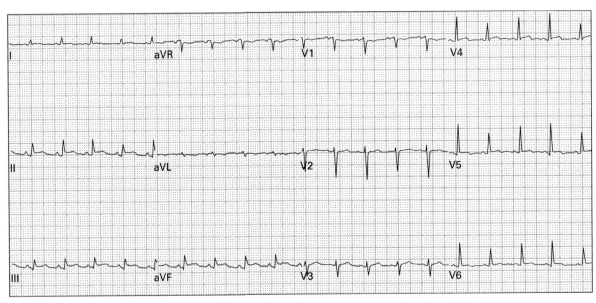

176. 32 year old man with pleuritic chest pain and dyspnea

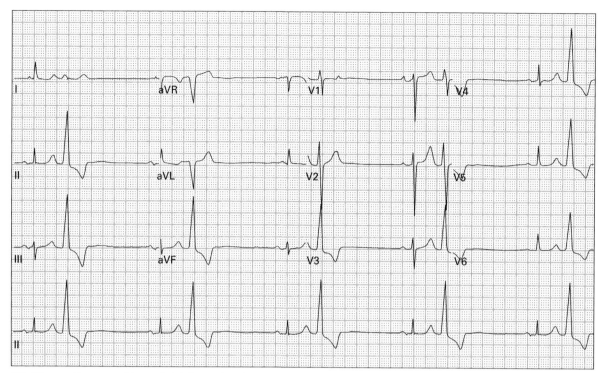

177. 95 year old woman with new facial droop, slurred speech, and hemiparesis

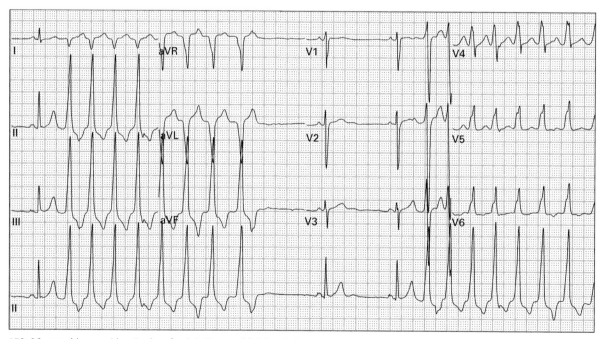

178. 36 year old man with episodes of palpitations and lightheadedness

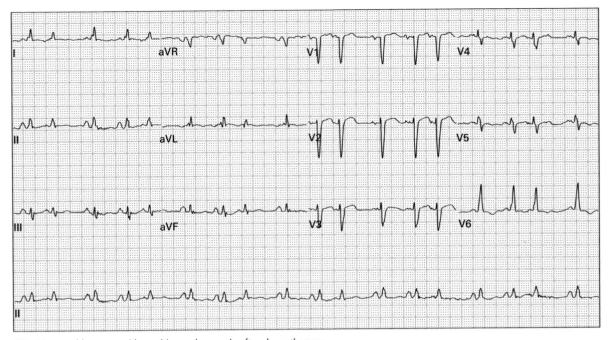

179. 70 year old woman with vomiting and anorexia after chemotherapy

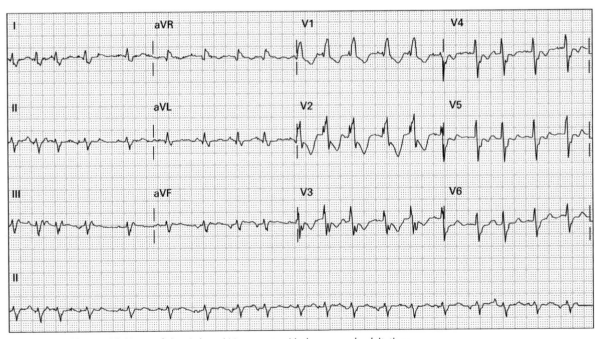

180. 60 year old man with history of chronic bronchitis presents with dyspnea and palpitations

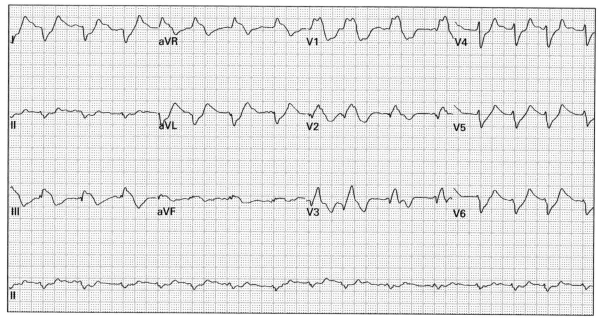

181. 63 year old woman with history of diabetes presents after a syncopal episode; she has been on non-steroidal anti-inflammatory medications for one month due to a back injury

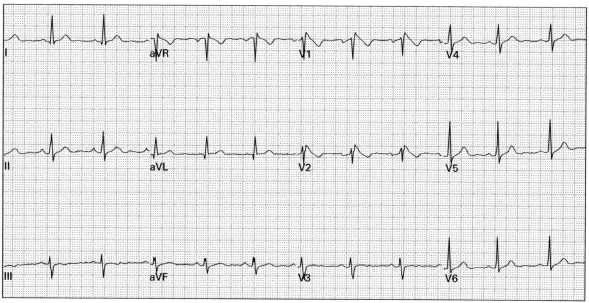

182. 54 year old woman presents after a syncopal episode

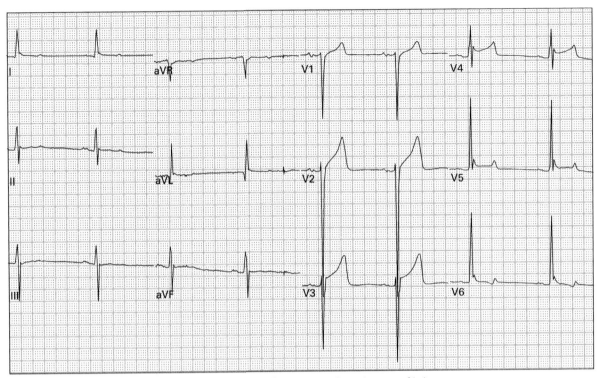

183. 71 year old man was sent to the emergency department from a nursing home because of lethargy

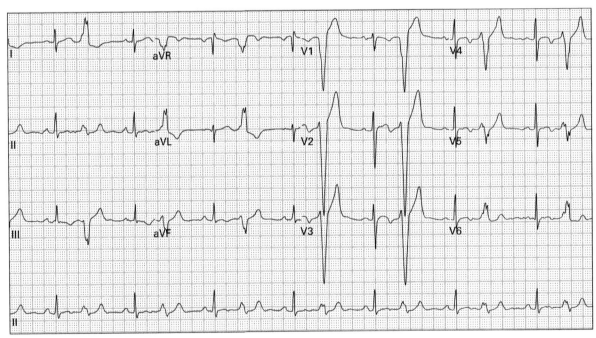

184. 35 year old man with chest pain and palpitations

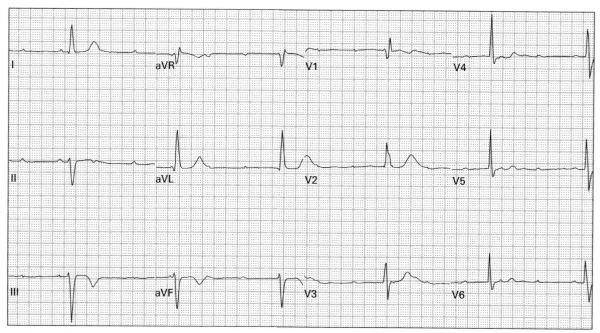

185. 50 year old man with chest pressure and extreme lightheadedness

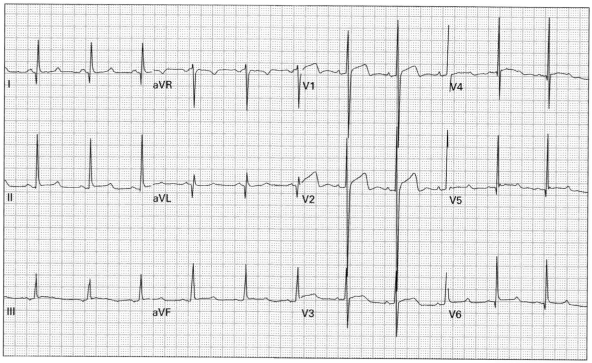

186. 29 year old man with a 30-minute episode of severe lightheadedness and palpitations after mild exertion

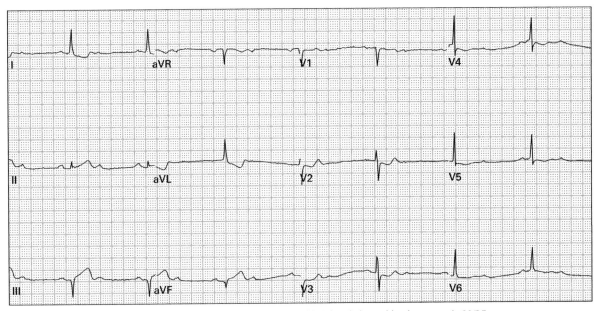

187. 62 year old man with epigastric burning, nausea, diaphoresis, and lightheadedness; blood pressure is 80/35

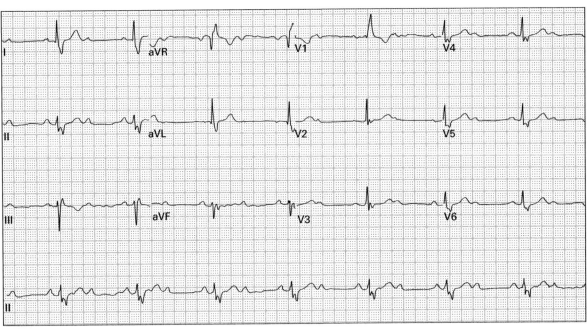

188. 68 year old woman with chest and throat discomfort

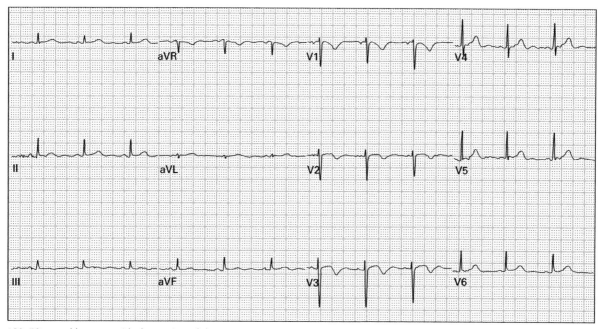

189. 78 year old woman with chest pain and dyspnea

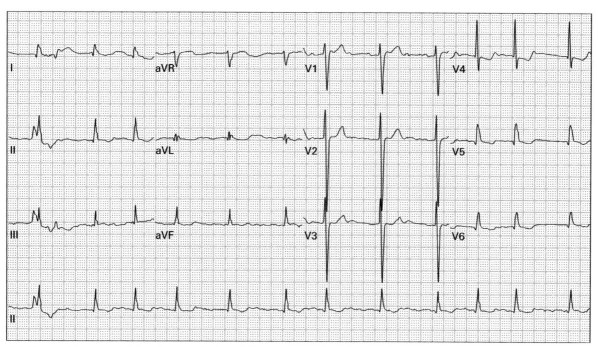

190. 67 year old woman with chronic congestive heart failure presents with weakness and vomiting

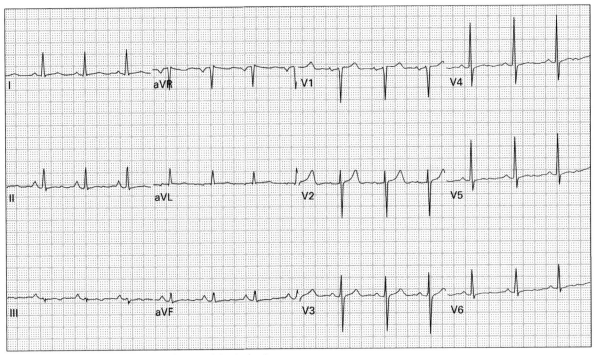

191. 46 year old woman with chest and upper abdominal pain

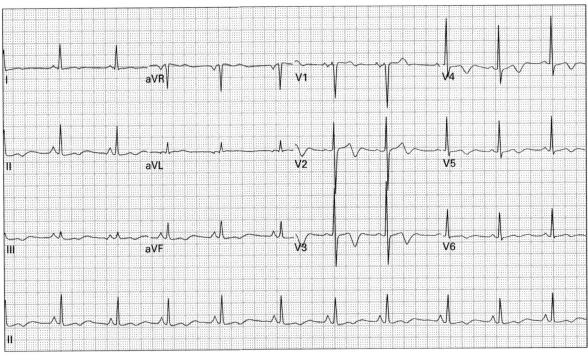

192. 46 year old woman with chest pain, upper abdominal pain, and diaphoresis

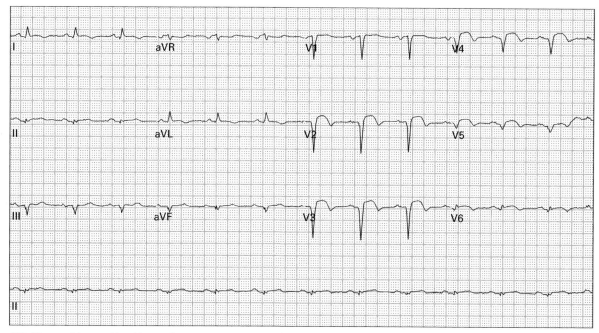

193. 73 year old man with a history of a recent MI presents with vomiting and diarrhea

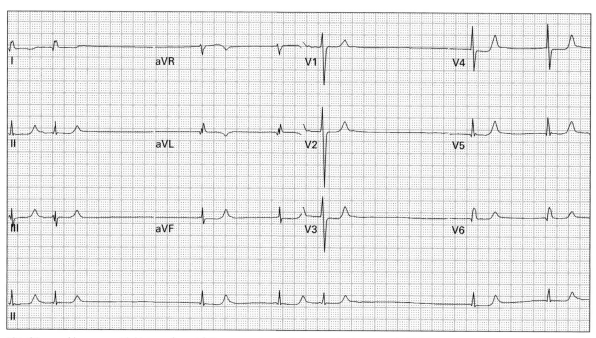

194. 67 year old woman with history of renal failure presents with lethargy; blood pressure is 75/35

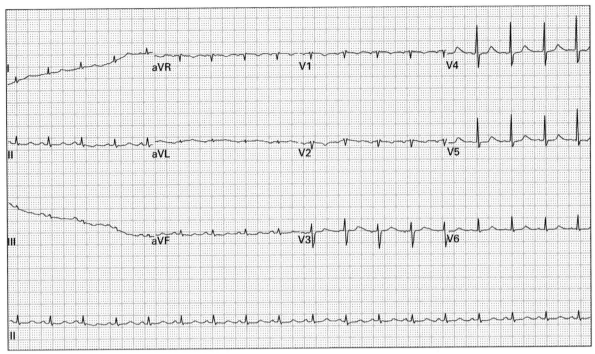

195. 39 year old man with end-stage acquired immunodeficiency syndrome (AIDS) presents with fever, dyspnea, and chest pressure; blood pressure is 90/35

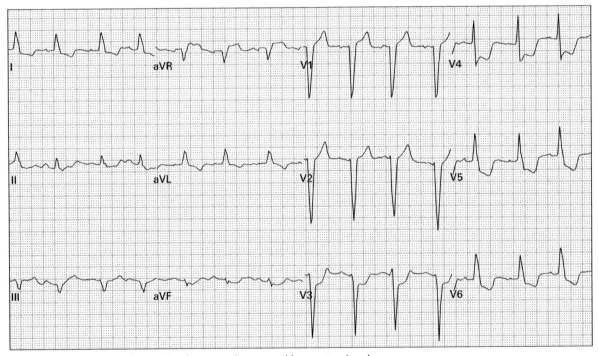

196. 81 year old woman with worsening dyspnea, orthopnea, and lower extremity edema

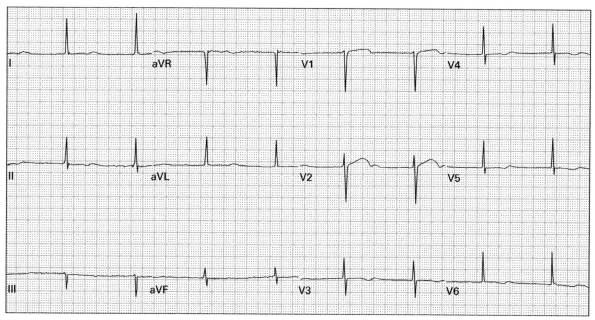

197. 57 year old woman with severe lightheadedness one day after beginning a new blood pressure medication

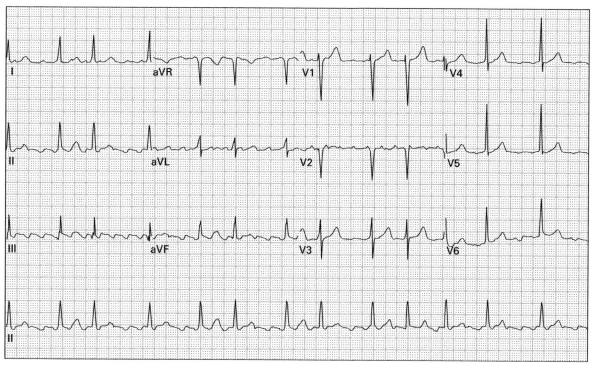

198. 69 year old woman with palpitations

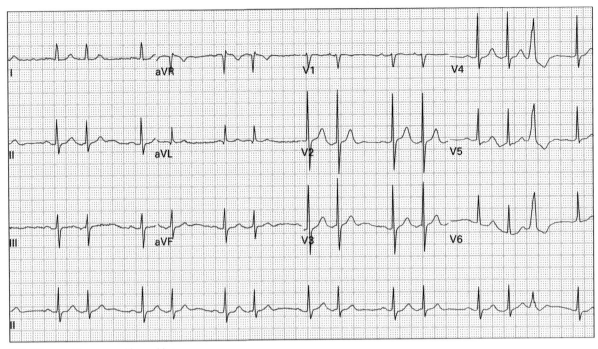

199. 95 year old woman with vomiting

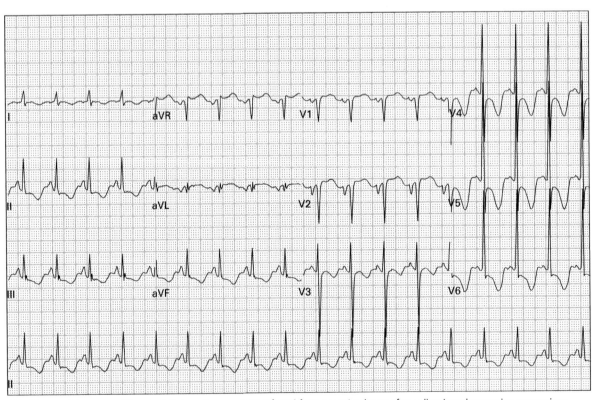

200. 54 year old woman with metastatic breast cancer is transferred from a nursing home after collapsing; she remains unconscious

ECG interpretations and comments

(Rates refer to ventricular rates unless otherwise specified; axis refers to QRS axis unless otherwise specified)

101.   **SR, acute inferior and right ventricular MI, low voltage.** ST-segment elevation and prominent wide ("hyperacute") T-waves indicate the early stages of an acute inferior MI. Reciprocal ST-segment depression in acute inferior MI is typical in leads I, aVL, and right precordial. In this case, however, ST-segment elevation is present in lead V1 and ST-segment depression is present in lead V2. This finding is highly specific for acute right ventricular infarction. Other findings on the 12-lead ECG which should suggest to the emergency physician the presence of right ventricular extension of inferior MI include the following:

- if the magnitude of ST-segment elevation in lead V1 exceeds the magnitude of ST-segment elevation in lead V2
- if the ST-segment in lead V1 is isoelectric and the ST-segment in lead V2 is significantly depressed
- if the magnitude of ST-segment elevation in lead III exceeds the magnitude of ST-segment elevation in lead II.

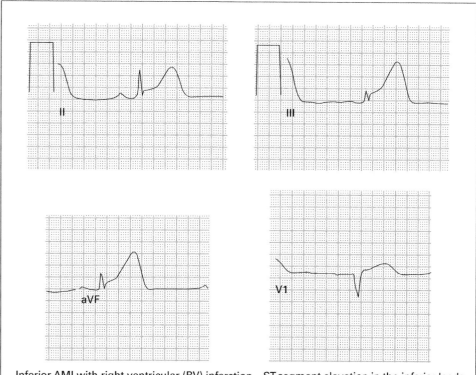

Inferior AMI with right ventricular (RV) infarction – ST-segment elevation in the inferior leads (II, III, and aVF), consistent with inferior wall AMI. Note that the magnitude of ST-segment elevation is minimal in all three leads, a finding noted not infrequently in inferior wall AMI. Right ventricular infarction is suggested by more pronounced ST-segment elevation in lead III (as compared to the ST-segment elevation in leads II and aVF) as well as ST-segment elevation in lead V1, the only lead of the standard 12-lead ECG which directly images the right ventricle

This figure also corresponds to case #101. These are additional ECGs to reinforce the point

Determination of ST-segment morphology

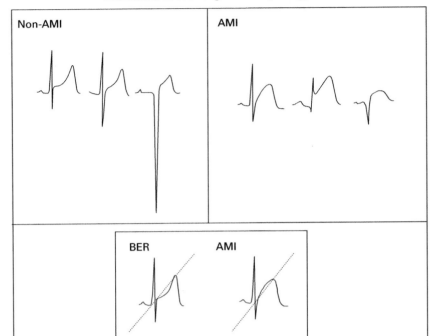

ST-segment elevation in AMI – the initial, upsloping portion of the ST-segment–T-wave complex is concave ("sagging downward") most often in non-AMI causes of ST-segment elevation, such as benign early repolarization. This morphology is compared to the flattened or convex pattern ("bulging upward") observed in the AMI patient. This morphologic observation is a very useful tool in "ruling in" AMI in chest pain patients with ST-segment elevation. Similar to many tools in clinical medicine, this electrocardiogrphic tool should only be used as a guideline. As with most guidelines, it is not infallible; patients with ST-segment elevation due to AMI may demonstrate *transient* concavity of this portion of the waveform, as seen in this case example.

The elevated ST-segment morphology may be determined by drawing a line from the J point to the apex of the T-wave: concave morphologies are noted when the ST-segment falls below the line while concave morphologies are demonstrated when the ST-segment is above the line

Right ventricular MI can be confirmed by performing an ECG using right-sided chest leads (see cases #30–31) or with bedside echocardiography. The presence of right ventricular extension of inferior MI is associated with increased morbidity and mortality. Preload-reducing medications (for example nitrates) should be used with caution, if at all, in patients with right ventricular MI. Low voltage in this case was caused by the patient's obesity and was evident on prior ECGs as well.

102. **SR, rate 69, LVH, intermittent WPW.** The amplitudes and morphologies of the QRS complexes change within each lead. These changes are clues that some type of abnormal ventricular conduction is occurring on an intermittent basis. Close inspection reveals that the second, fifth, eighth, and ninth QRS complexes are associated with the classic triad of WPW: short PR-segments, slightly wider QRS complexes, and delta-waves.

103. **SR, rate 82, prolonged QT.** The QT-interval appears prolonged because of a large, "camel-hump" type of T-wave. This type of T-wave should prompt consideration of two possibilities:

- a "buried" P-wave has caused the deformity in the T-wave
- the second "hump" is actually a U-wave that has fused to the end of the T-wave (referred to as "T-U fusion").

T-U fusion is common in cases of moderate or severe hypokalemia. Some authors do not consider hypokalemia a cause of prolonged QT-interval because the wide T-wave is actually the result of a T-U fusion complex. This patient's serum potassium was 3·0 mEq/L (normal 3·5–5·3 mEq/L).

104. **SR, rate 97, incomplete RBBB, T-wave abnormality consistent with inferior and anteroseptal ischemia.** The prominent inverted T-waves in the precordial leads should prompt consideration of a large proximal LAD obstructing lesion. The T-wave inversions in this condition are often referred to as "Wellens' waves" or Wellens' sign. However, the presence of a rightward axis, incomplete RBBB, and simultaneous T-wave inversions in the inferior and anteroseptal leads points to an alternative deadly diagnosis – massive pulmonary embolism. The prominent upright P-wave in lead V1 is also typical of large pulmonary embolism. This patient was treated in the emergency department with intravenous heparin. However, he developed respiratory arrest and died despite resuscitative efforts. Earlier consideration had been given to empiric thrombolytic therapy but was withheld because of known metastases to the brain. Autopsy confirmed the presence of multiple pulmonary emboli including a saddle embolus.

105. **ST with frequent PACs in a pattern of atrial trigeminy, rate 115, PRWP, RAE, non-specific T-wave flattening in lateral leads.** Close inspection of the ECG reveals a regularly irregular rhythm; the QRS complexes occur in groups of three. The first and second QRS complex in each group are preceded by large P-waves, but the third QRS complex in each group is preceded by a smaller P-wave that occurs prematurely – a PAC. In this case, all of the PACs are conducted to the ventricle and therefore are followed by QRS complexes. However, if the PAC occurs too early in the cycle and the ventricle has not yet "reset," the atrial impulse will not be conducted and will result in a pause in the rhythm. This frequently leads to a misdiagnosis of second degree AV block. Examples of this will follow.

106. **ST with second degree AV block with 2:1 AV conduction, rate 75, PRWP.** The rhythm was initially misdiagnosed as SR because non-conducted P-waves are not obvious in most leads. However, close inspection of all 12 leads reveals non-conducted P-waves, best seen in leads V2 and V3. The P-waves occur in a regular rhythm at a rate of 150/minute. When interpreting the ECG rhythm, one should never rely exclusively on lead II (the most common lead provided as a rhythm strip); **all 12 leads** must be evaluated carefully. PRWP in this case was due to a prior anteroseptal MI.

107. **ST, rate 128, LAE, non-specific intraventricular conduction delay.** The ECG demonstrates findings highly suggestive of cyclic antidepressant overdose:
      - tachycardia
      - rightward axis
      - R-wave amplitude in aVR ≥3 mm
      - slight prolongation of the QRS-interval (intraventricular conduction delay).

Another ECG finding commonly found in cases of cyclic antidepressant toxicity is prolongation of the QT-interval, although the interval is normal in this case. All of these abnormalities resolve with treatment. Cyclic antidepressants are an important part of the differential diagnosis for rightward axis, QRS-interval prolongation, and QT-interval prolongation. The patient in this case later admitted that he had tried to commit suicide by overdosing on amitriptyline, a tricyclic antidepressant medication. Emergency physicians should be familiar with the differential diagnosis of common medication overdoses that produce tachycardia: sympathomimetics (for example amphetamines, cocaine, over-the-counter decongestants), anticholinergics (for example cyclic antidepressants, antihistamines), and methylxanthines (for example theophylline, caffeine).

108. **SR, rate 79, incomplete RBBB, T-wave abnormality consistent with anteroseptal ischemia, non-specific T-wave abnormality in inferior leads.** The ECG is suggestive of pulmonary embolism. An incomplete RBBB pattern is present, suggesting the presence of right ventricular dilatation (strain). T-wave abnormalities are common in pulmonary embolism. Simultaneous T-wave inversions in the inferior and anteroseptal leads, as discussed previously, are highly specific for pulmonary embolism; however, T-wave inversions isolated to the anteroseptal leads have greater sensitivity. Note that this patient is not tachycardic. Tachycardia is present in fewer than half of patients with pulmonary embolism.

109. **Atrial tachycardia with variable AV block, rate 70; rhythm suggestive of digoxin toxicity.** The atrial rate is 200/minute, generally referred to as atrial **tachycardia** (or "paroxysmal" atrial tachycardia, PAT). Atrial **flutter** is diagnosed when the atrial rate is 250–350/minute. Varying degrees of AV conduction are present, producing a ventricular rate of approximately 70/minute. PAT with variable block is one of the common dysrhythmias present in the setting of digoxin toxicity. This patient's serum digoxin level was 4·4 ng/ml (normal 0·5–2·2 ng/ml).

110. **ST, rate 130, low voltage.** Low voltage is diagnosed when the amplitudes of the QRS complexes in all the limb leads are less than 5 mm or when the amplitudes of the QRS complexes in all the precordial leads are less than 10 mm. The differential diagnosis of low QRS voltage is extensive; it includes myxedema, large pericardial effusion, large pleural effusion, end-stage cardiomyopathy, severe chronic obstructive pulmonary disease, severe obesity, infiltrative myocardial diseases, constrictive pericarditis, and prior massive MI. However, the combination of low voltage plus tachycardia should always prompt strong consideration of large pericardial effusion and potential pericardial tamponade. The patient in this case did have echocardiographic evidence of pericardial tamponade (right ventricular diastolic collapse). Emergent pericardiotomy was performed and the patient did well.

111. **SR, rate 75, LVH, incomplete RBBB with ST-segment elevation in right precordial leads consistent with the Brugada syndrome.** The Brugada syndrome was first described by Brugada[1] in 1992 as a frequent cause of sudden death in patients with structurally normal hearts. The syndrome is characterized by ECG abnormalities in leads V1–V3 and development of polymorphic or monomorphic VT (causing sudden death if persistent, syncope if self-terminating). The ECG abnormalities in leads V1–V3 consist of an RBBB or incomplete RBBB pattern as well as ST-segment elevation. The ST-segment elevation is often of an convex-upwards morphology, although in this case the less common concave-upwards ST-segment elevation is present. Definitive diagnosis is made during electrophysiology studies, as was the case with this patient. Emergency physicians should become familiar with the Brugada syndrome and promptly refer suspected patients for electrophysiologic studies. The only effective treatment is placement of an internal cardioverter-defibrillator (ICD). Without placement of an ICD, mortality is approximately 10%/year.[2]

112. **SR with second degree AV block type 1 (Mobitz I, Wenckebach), frequent PVCs in a pattern of ventricular trigeminy, rate 73, non-specific T-wave flattening in inferior leads.** The rhythm is regularly irregular with groups of three QRS complexes. The first two QRS complexes in each group are narrow-complex and are preceded by P-waves. The third QRS complex in each group is a PVC; thus, ventricular trigeminy is diagnosed. Mobitz I AV conduction is identified based on the presence of regular P-waves with PR-segment lengthening from the first to the second beat in each cycle. Non-conducted P-waves are obscured by the PVCs.

113. **ST, rate 110, acute PMI.** ST-segment depression in the right precordial leads is usually associated with one of three possible conditions:
    - acute anteroseptal myocardial ischemia
    - reciprocal change associated with acute inferior MI
    - PMI.

The presence of prominent R-waves and upright T-waves in these same leads indicates the diagnosis is PMI. Most PMIs occur in association with inferior MI, and a lesser number occur in association with lateral MI. Less than 5% are isolated PMI, as was the case here. Confirmation can be accomplished by placement of posterior leads (place leads V5 and V6 inferolateral and inferomedial to the inferior tip of the scapula) and evaluating for the "usual" signs of acute MI (ST-segment elevation, inverted T-waves, Q-waves) in these leads.

114. **SR with sinus arrhythmia, rate 77, acute septal MI.** ST-segment elevation in lead V1 is associated with several conditions:
- acute anteroseptal MI
- acute right ventricular MI
- Brugada syndrome
- LVH
- LBBB
- pulmonary embolism.

The presence of reciprocal ST-segment depression in other leads is highly specific for acute MI. Acute right ventricular MI is unlikely because of the absence of evidence of acute inferior MI, which almost always accompanies right ventricular MI. ST-segment elevation is also noted in lead aVR. In the setting of acute MI, ST-segment elevation in lead aVR indicates proximal obstruction of the LAD or left main coronary artery. When the amplitude of ST-segment elevation in lead aVR is ≥1·5 mm, the prognosis is poor, with mortality rates as high as 75%.[3]

115. **SR with sinus arrhythmia, rate 73, acute inferior and right ventricular MI.** Right ventricular MI is suggested on the standard 12-lead ECG when:
- ST-segment elevation is present in lead V1 and ST-segment depression is present in lead V2
- ST-segment elevation is present in both leads V1 and V2 but the magnitude of ST-segment elevation in lead V1 exceeds the magnitude of ST-segment elevation in lead V2
- the ST-segment in lead V1 is isoelectric and the ST-segment in lead V2 is significantly depressed
- the magnitude of ST-segment elevation in lead III exceeds the magnitude of ST-segment elevation in lead II.

In this case, right ventricular MI is suggested by criteria #3 and #4 above.

116. **SR, rate 75, previous inferior MI, inversion of electrodes V1 and V3.** Prominent R-waves in lead V1 (defined as an R:S ratio ≥1) exist as a normal variant in only 1% of patients.[4] Therefore, emergency physicians should be familiar with the potential causes of this ECG finding: WPW, PMI, RBBB (or incomplete RBBB), ventricular ectopy, RVH, acute right ventricular dilatation (right ventricular "strain," for example massive pulmonary embolism), hypertrophic cardiomyopathy, progressive muscular dystrophy, dextrocardia, and misplaced precordial electrodes. In this case, electrodes V1 and V3 were inadvertently switched in position, producing the prominent R-wave in lead V1. The normal ECG demonstrates gradual enlargement of the R-wave and decreasing size of the S-wave across the precordium. Loss of this proper R-wave and S-wave progression should lead to suspicion of misplaced leads. Another clue is that the P-wave in lead V1 usually is inverted, flat, or biphasic and is upright in leads V2–V6. In this case, the P-wave in lead V3 is flat but upright in lead V1.

117. **SB with first degree AV block and frequent non-conducted PACs in a pattern of atrial trigeminy, rate 37, bifascicular block (RBBB and LAFB), LAE, LVH.** This type of rhythm is frequently misdiagnosed as second degree AV block type 2 (Mobitz II) because of the presence of non-conducted P-waves and a constant PR-interval in the P-waves that **are** conducted. The key finding that excludes the diagnosis of Mobitz II, however, is that the non-conducted P-waves **occur early in the rhythm** (the PP-interval should be constant

in second degree AV block), i.e, they are simply PACs. Non-conducted (or "blocked") PACs are a common cause of pauses on the ECG rhythm strip. When a PAC occurs **too** early in the cycle and the ventricle has not had enough time to "reset," the atrial beat will fail to produce ventricular depolarization. The PAC causes the sinus node to reset; therefore there is a delay before the next sinus P-wave occurs. The result is a pause on the ECG rhythm strip. It is advisable to always use ECG calipers and rule out the possibility of non-conducted PACs anytime second degree AV block is considered. The distinction is critical; second degree AV block may need treatment with a pacemaker, whereas non-conducted PACs rarely need treatment at all. In this case, the patient did have some electrolyte abnormalities which, when corrected, resulted in resolution of the PACs and a normal ventricular rate and rhythm. Atrial bigeminy is diagnosed when every second atrial complex is a PAC; atrial trigeminy is diagnosed when every third atrial complex is a PAC, etc.

118. **AV junctional tachycardia, rate 115, incomplete RBBB, acute anterior MI, inferior MI of uncertain age.** There is no evidence of normal atrial activity, leading to the diagnosis of an AV junctional rhythm. Small retrograde P-waves are noted following the QRS complexes in leads I and aVL. ST-segment elevation in the anterior leads, even in the presence of incomplete or full RBBB is considered reliable evidence of acute injury. Q-waves in the inferior and anterior leads indicate transmural infarction. However, the inferior leads show no evidence of acute ST-segment or T-wave abnormality, so it is difficult to be certain whether the inferior MI is recent or old. Review of prior ECGs later confirmed that the inferior MI had occurred several years earlier.

119. **Atrial fibrillation with slow ventricular response, rate 40.** The underlying atrial rhythm shows a fine fibrillatory pattern, consistent with the patient's prior history of atrial fibrillation. Atrial fibrillation is usually associated with a ventricular response rate of 120–170/minute; slower ventricular response rates indicate severe AV nodal disease, hypothermia, or medication effects. The history in this patient indicates overmedication, and the most likely cause is toxicity from digoxin, a calcium channel blocking medication (CCB), or a beta-receptor blocking medication (BB). In the bradycardic patient with chronic atrial fibrillation, the distinction between CCB toxicity versus BB toxicity on the ECG is extremely difficult. However, digoxin toxicity usually reveals some helpful clues: occasional PVCs, the "hockey stick" appearance of the terminal portion of the R-wave (also referred to by some as the "Salvadore Dali moustache" appearance), and complete heart block with a regular junctional or ventricular escape rhythm. None of these clues to digoxin toxicity are present. This patient had recently been given a new prescription for a higher dose of a calcium channel blocking medication but continued taking the previous-dose pills as well. He was treated with intravenous calcium and did well.

120. **Atrial flutter, rate 113, RBBB.** The most important causes of a wide-complex irregular rhythm have previously been discussed: atrial fibrillation with aberrant conduction (for example bundle branch block), atrial fibrillation with WPW, and PVT. However, two other entities that are somewhat less common (and less deadly) should be mentioned as well: atrial flutter with variable block and aberrant conduction and MAT with aberrant conduction. As with the narrow-complex irregular rhythms, the diagnosis is made by scrutinizing the ECG for atrial activity. In this case, the answer is found in lead V1 which demonstrates flutter-waves. Notice that lead II, which is usually the rhythm strip provided by most ECG machines, is not helpful. Lead V1 is often the best lead for identifying atrial activity.

121. **SB with second degree AV block type 1 (Mobitz I, Wenckebach), rate 58, LVH with repolarization abnormality and non-specific intraventricular conduction delay, PRWP.** This is a case of very slowly progressing Mobitz I conduction. Many of the P-waves are hidden by, or "buried within," the T-waves, increasing the difficulty of interpretation. The PP-interval remains constant, typical of second degree AV block. Inverted T-waves in the lateral leads are not uncommon in LVH and are due to abnormal repolarization. The inverted T-waves associated with LVH should be asymmetric and should not be present in the right precordial leads. LVH can sometimes produce slight QRS-interval prolongation, seen here, due to an intraventricular conduction delay.

122. **SR, rate 60, high left ventricular voltage, abnormal Q-waves in lateral leads suggestive of hypertrophic cardiomyopathy (HCM).** HCM, also known as idiopathic hypertrophic subaortic stenosis (IHSS), hypertrophic obstructive cardiomyopathy (HOCM), and asymmetric septal hypertrophy (ASH), is a frequent cause of sudden death in adolescents and young adults. Characteristic ECG findings include:
    - large-amplitude QRS complexes
    - deep narrow Q-waves in the inferior and/or lateral leads, mimicking inferior and/or lateral MI
    - tall R-waves in leads V1–V2 that mimic PMI or RVH.

    Any or all of these ECG abnormalities may be found and are attributed to ventricular septal hypertrophy. Perhaps the most specific finding is the appearance of the deep narrow Q-waves. They are often mistaken for MI-type Q-waves, but they tend to be deeper and more narrow. Definitive diagnosis of HCM is made with doppler echocardiography. Although this patient meets the usual voltage criteria for LVH, the term "high left ventricular voltage" (HLVV) is often preferred in patients under the age of 40 with large-amplitude QRS complexes. "LVH" implies the existence of an abnormal condition; on the contrary, many normal healthy adolescents and young adults manifest large-amplitude QRS complexes on ECG. HLVV has a poor correlation with echocardiographic evidence of LVH in young patients.

123. **SR, rate 60, RAE, LVH, T-wave abnormality and prolonged QT-interval consistent with anteroseptal ischemia versus hypokalemia.** RAE is diagnosed based on the P-wave amplitude >2·5 mm in the inferior leads. The T-wave morphology, initial portion inverted and the terminal portion upright, as well as the markedly prolonged QT-interval (QT-interval 0·624 seconds, QTc-interval 0·613 seconds) suggests the presence of a T-wave–U-wave fusion complex. The patient was initially thought to have acute anterior ischemia with Wellens' sign (biphasic T-waves in the mid-precordial leads, highly specific for a large proximal obstructing LAD lesion). However, the biphasic Wellens' T-waves have an initial upright component followed by an inverted terminal component. The serum potassium level in this patient was 2·3 mEq/L (normal 3·5–5·3 mEq/L).

124. **Multifocal atrial tachycardia (MAT) with occasional PVCs, rate 110, PRWP.** The differential diagnosis of a narrow-complex irregular tachycardia includes atrial fibrillation, atrial flutter with variable block, and MAT. The presence of distinct P-waves excludes the diagnosis of atrial fibrillation. On the contrary, there are at least three different types of P-waves (in terms of morphology) that occur at irregular intervals, confirming the diagnosis of MAT and excluding the diagnosis of atrial flutter. MAT is often associated with pulmonary disease. This patient was suffering from an exacerbation of emphysema. Leftward axis, present in this case, is a common finding in patients with severe emphysema.

125. **SR, rate 70, LAE, acute anterolateral MI, non-specific T-wave flattening in inferior leads.** Without the knowledge of any history or the availability of an old ECG, the above interpretation would have to be made. This patient, however, has no cardiopulmonary symptoms and the ECG was done purely as an admission protocol. She does have a history of a prior MI. All of this information strongly suggests the presence of a left ventricular aneurysm (LVA). An old ECG was obtained and demonstrated similar findings. LVAs are associated with Q-waves and persistent ST-segment elevation even though acute ischemia has resolved. The ECG abnormalities remain indefinitely. Most, but not all, LVAs occur on the anterior wall of the left ventricle, producing the persistent ST-segment elevation in the precordial leads. One helpful (though not perfect) clue to distinguish LVAs from acute MIs is that LVAs are **not** associated with reciprocal ST-segment depression in other leads.

126. **SR with occasional premature supraventricular complexes, rate 96, LVH, RBBB, acute anterolateral MI, inferior MI of uncertain age.** The rhythm is regular in the initial portion of the ECG, but premature complexes interrupt the rhythm in the latter portion. The 11th and 15th QRS complexes occur early and are preceded by small P-waves – PACs. The 12th QRS complex, however, has no clearly defined preceding P-wave

and may therefore represent either a PAC (with the P-wave buried in the preceding T-wave) or a premature AV junctional complex (PJC). A PVC is unlikely, given the similar morphology of the QRS complex to the other QRS complexes. Acute anterolateral MI is diagnosed based on the presence of ST-segment elevation in leads V3–V6. ST-segment elevation should always be considered abnormal in the precordial leads in RBBB. Q-waves are present in the inferior leads, but there are no associated ST-segment or T-wave abnormalities, suggesting that the inferior infarction is old. An ECG from two years earlier confirmed that the inferior MI was old, but the anterolateral MI was acute.

127. **Atrial flutter with variable block, rate 90, bifascicular block (RBBB and LAFB).** The rhythm was initially misdiagnosed as atrial fibrillation because of the irregularity of the rhythm and the absence of obvious atrial activity on the lead II rhythm strip. Close inspection of all 12 leads, however, shows distinct flutter-waves in lead V1.

128. **SR with intermittent first degree AV block and LBBB, T-wave abnormality consistent with inferior and lateral ischemia.** The underlying rhythm appears to be SR with rate 73/minute, present during the initial and final portions of the ECG. The middle portion of the ECG displays SR with first degree AV block and LBBB with rate 94/minute. The presence of the first degree AV block and the LBBB are likely acceleration-dependent (rate-dependent). Bundle branch blocks can also be deceleration-dependent (occurring in the presence of bradycardia).

129. **SB versus AV junctional rhythm, rate 51, prolonged QT-interval, J-waves consistent with hypothermia, non-specific T-wave flattening in inferior leads.** Artifact (due to patient shivering) obscures any atrial activity; therefore, it is difficult to distinguish between SB and AV junctional rhythm. The QT-interval is prolonged (QT-interval 0·608 seconds, QTc-interval 0·560 seconds) and should prompt consideration of the causes of QT-interval prolongation: hypokalemia, hypomagnesemia, hypocalcemia, acute myocardial ischemia, elevated intracranial pressure, drugs with sodium channel blocking effects (for example cyclic antidepressants, quinidine, etc.), hypothermia, and congenital prolonged QT syndrome. J-waves ("Osborne waves") are present in the anterior and lateral precordial leads. Although not pathognomonic for

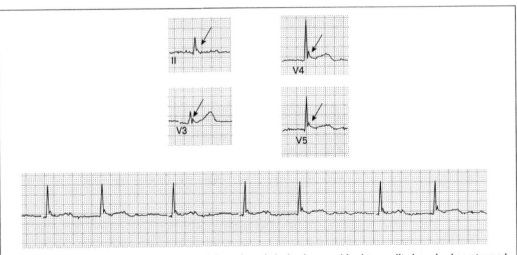

The most common ECG finding in patients with hypothermia is the J wave; this abnormality has also been termed the "Osborne wave." This finding (arrow) is characterized as a positive deflection in the terminal portion of the QRS complex and elevation of the J point. J waves are most commonly found in the anterior and lateral precordial leads and in lead II, although they may be present in only a single lead. They usually occur in patients with core body temperatures less than 32°C (90°F) and often appear larger when the temperature is below 30°C (86°F). The size of the J waves usually correlates inversely with the body temperature; as the body temperature increases, the J wave gradually becomes smaller. Other findings suggestive of hypothermia in this example include the motion (tremor) artifact and slow ventricular rate hypothermia, J-waves are highly sensitive and specific for hypothermia. This patient's rectal temperature was 28·5 degrees Celsius (83·3 degrees Fahrenheit).

130. **Atrial tachycardia with variable AV block, rate 40, previous inferior MI; rhythm suggestive of digoxin toxicity.** This rhythm is often referred to as paroxysmal atrial tachycardia (PAT) with block. Atrial activity with a rate of 214/minute is clearly present in most leads. Although the atrial rhythm has a flutter or "sawtooth" pattern, the term "flutter" is usually reserved for atrial rates >250/minute. PAT with block generally is believed to occur due to increased automaticity in the atrium as well as impaired conduction in the AV node, leading to high grades of AV block and relatively slow ventricular rates. Digoxin toxicity is the most common cause of PAT with block and was the cause of this patient's symptoms.

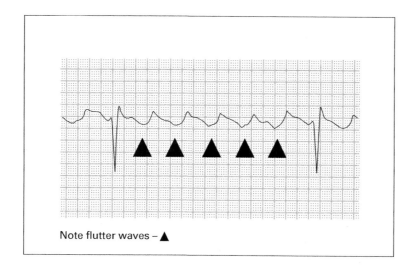

Note flutter waves – ▲

131. **SR with sinus arrhythmia, rate 74, incomplete RBBB with ST-segment elevation in right precordial leads consistent with the Brugada syndrome.** The Brugada syndrome, as discussed in case #111, is associated with ECG abnormalities consisting of an incomplete or complete RBBB pattern with ST-segment elevation in leads V1–V3 (although occasionally only evident in leads V1–V2). Patients with the Brugada syndrome are predisposed to the development of polymorphic (more common) or monomorphic VT, leading to sudden death. If the dysrhythmia aborts spontaneously, the patient will report a syncopal episode. The **only** effective treatment is placement of an internal cardioverter-defibrillator. Mortality otherwise is 10%/year, highlighting the importance of early recognition and referral to an electrophysiologist. See figure on p. 138.

132. **SR with second degree AV block type 2 (Mobitz II), rate 48, LBBB.** The majority of the ECG rhythm demonstrates second degree AV block with 2:1 conduction. It is very difficult to be certain whether these 2:1 rhythms are Mobitz I or Mobitz II. However in this case, there is a single area in the mid-portion of the ECG in which 3:2 conduction is present, and the PR-interval remains constant in this area. The constant PR-interval confirms the diagnosis of Mobitz II.

133. **SR with AV dissociation and third degree AV block, AV junctional rhythm, rate 50, LBBB.** Once again, lead V1 is the best lead for identification of atrial activity on this ECG. Independent atrial and ventricular activity (AV dissociation) is identified by the presence of varying PR-intervals. There is no indication that any of the P-waves are conducted to the ventricle; therefore third degree AV block is diagnosed. The QRS complexes are wide. This may be due to a ventricular escape rhythm or an AV junctional escape rhythm with aberrant ventricular conduction (for example bundle branch block). The rate (50/minute) is suggestive of an AV junctional rhythm, and the morphology of the QRS complexes is consistent with an LBBB pattern. Comparison with previous ECGs confirmed that the patient did have a pre-existent LBBB with identical QRS morphologies.

This figure corresponds to case #131. Brugada syndrome

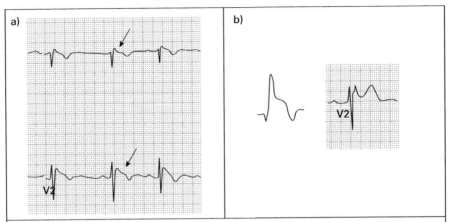

a) The "coved" type ST-segment elevation (arrow) from the ECG case – note the convex morphology. b) A comparison of the two types of ST-segment morphology in the Brugada syndrome: LEFT – the "coved" type ST-segment elevation (note the convex morphology); RIGHT – "saddle" type ST-segment elevation (note the concave morphology)

134. **SB with second degree AV block type 1 (Mobitz I, Wenckebach), rate 47.** Artifact obscures the rhythm interpretation in most of the leads, but P-waves can be seen well in the lead II rhythm strip. Subtle progressive lengthening of the PR-interval occurs prior to the non-conducted P-wave. The changing PR-interval can best be appreciated by comparing the PR-interval preceding the non-conducted P-wave with the PR-interval that follows.

135. **Atrial flutter with variable AV block, rate 116, LVH with non-specific intraventricular conduction delay and repolarization abnormality.** The rhythm was initially misdiagnosed as atrial fibrillation because of the irregularity of the rhythm. However, the R-R interval is constant within groups of beats, uncharacteristic of atrial fibrillation. In addition, close inspection of all leads reveals the presence of atrial complexes (rate 300/minute) in leads V1 and V2, confirming the diagnosis of atrial flutter. The QRS complexes are slightly wide (0·112 seconds), due to a non-specific intraventricular conduction delay often found with LVH. Inverted T-waves in the lateral leads are often associated with LVH as well and are due to abnormal repolarization.

136. **Atrial fibrillation with WPW, rate 152.** The presence of a wide-complex irregular rhythm should prompt consideration of atrial fibrillation with aberrant conduction (usually bundle branch block), atrial fibrillation with WPW, and polymorphic VT (PVT). The QRS complexes show marked variation in morphology, essentially excluding the diagnosis of atrial fibrillation with bundle branch block. Atrial fibrillation with WPW is characterized by an significant variation in the QRS complex morphology; rates can approach 250–300/minute is some portions of the ECG, whereas rates in other areas of the ECG are often <200/minute. In contrast, PVT tends to be associated with ventricular rates that are persistently rapid and often in excess of 300/minute (see case #89). This patient was hemodynamically stable, so she was treated with intravenous procainamide and converted back to SR. See figure on p. 139.

137. **AV junctional rhythm, rate 53, RBBB, acute inferior MI.** The absence of P-waves and the wide-complex QRS complexes should prompt consideration of an AV junctional rhythm versus a ventricular rhythm. However, the QRS morphology (rsR' in lead V1, slightly wide S-waves in leads I and V6) and the ventricular rate between 40–60/minute strongly favors an AV junctional rhythm. The final QRS complex is narrow and is preceded by a P-wave, indicating occasional atrial activity that is conducted normally through the ventricle. Q-waves and ST-segment elevation in the inferior leads indicate acute infarction with persistent ischemia. ST-segment elevation in lead III that exceeds the magnitude of ST-segment elevation in lead II suggests right ventricular extension of the MI.

147. **SR with sinus arrhythmia, rate 75, prolonged QT.** The major abnormality found in this ECG is the markedly prolonged QT-interval (QT-interval 0·520 seconds, QTc-interval 0·581 seconds). Prolonged QT-interval is associated with hypokalemia, hypomagnesemia, hypocalcemia, acute myocardial ischemia, elevated intracranial pressure, drugs with sodium channel blocking effects (for example cyclic antidepressants, quinidine, etc.), hypothermia, and congenital prolonged QT syndrome. In this case, the abnormality was caused by an overdose of one of the patient's antipsychotic medications. These medications, as well as many others, are associated with the prolonged QT-interval and the potential for developing torsades de pointes.

148. **Underlying AV junctional rhythm with intermittent episodes of polymorphic VT, torsade de pointes (TDP).** This is the same patient as in case #147. Intermittent short runs of polymorphic VT have developed. Between each group of VT complexes is a single, narrow QRS-complex preceded by a P-wave. The P-waves in leads II and III are inverted, indicating an ectopic source of the P-waves; and the PR-interval is <0·12 seconds. These two findings strongly suggest that the source of the P-waves is the AV junction (AV junctional rhythm with retrograde P-waves). The presence of a pre-existent prolonged QT-interval allows this particular case of polymorphic VT to be referred to as TDP. Soon after this ECG was obtained, the patient developed sustained TDP. He was electrically cardioverted, treated with intravenous magnesium, and received appropriate treatment for his overdose.

149. **ST with AV dissociation and third degree AV block, AV junctional rhythm, rate 41, LBBB, non-specific T-wave abnormality.** Independent atrial (sinus rate 130) and ventricular activity exist, indicating AV dissociation. There do not appear to be any P-waves conducted to the ventricle, indicating third degree (complete) heart block. The wide QRS complexes can suggest a ventricular rhythm originating from within the ventricle itself; or they could represent an AV junctional rhythm conducted to the ventricles with an LBBB. The rate of 41 is consistent with **either** a ventricular rhythm or an AV junctional rhythm. The distinction is difficult, but a previous ECG was obtained in this case and showed evidence of a prior LBBB with similar QRS morphology.

150. **MAT, rate 124, LVH, non-specific T-wave flattening in inferior and lateral leads.** The main considerations when the rhythm is narrow-complex and irregular are atrial fibrillation, atrial flutter with variable block, and MAT. Distinction amongst these three diagnoses is based on scrutiny of the atrial activity. Atrial fibrillation will generally have absence of distinct atrial complexes; atrial flutter will have evidence of rapid **regular** atrial complexes, at least half of which will be non-conducted; and MAT will have **irregular** atrial complexes of at least three different morphologies, and there will be a 1:1 relationship between the atrial complexes and the QRS complexes (usually all will be conducted). This ECG shows all of the characteristics of MAT.

151. **ST with AV dissociation and third degree AV block, ventricular escape rhythm, rate 25, T-wave abnormality consistent with anterior ischemia, non-specific T-wave flattening in inferior leads.** ECG criteria for third degree AV block (complete heart block) are present; there is evidence of independent atrial and ventricular activity (the atrial rate is 100, the ventricular rate is 25), the PR-intervals vary randomly, and there is no evidence that any of the P-waves are conducted to the ventricles. Occasionally, AV dissociation (independent atrial and ventricular activity) may exist in the absence of complete heart block. In these cases, there will be ECG evidence of some P-waves being conducted to the ventricle.

152. **Atrial flutter with 2:1 AV conduction, rate 125, LBBB.** The rhythm is wide-complex and regular, prompting consideration of VT, SVT with aberrant conduction, and ST with aberrant conduction. A less common entity should be considered as well – atrial flutter with aberrant conduction. Both ST and atrial flutter are characterized by regular distinct atrial complexes, whereas VT and SVT are less likely to demonstrate regular distinct atrial complexes. In this case, atrial complexes are clearly found in lead V1 and led to the misdiagnosis of ST. One may notice, however, an irregular appearance to the T-wave in lead V1 – "a camel hump"

appearance. As discussed earlier, this type of irregular appearance of the T-wave should always prompt consideration of hypokalemia (T-U fusion complex) and "buried" P-waves. In this case, the irregular T-wave appearance was caused by the latter; the first "hump of the camel" is a buried P-wave, or flutter-wave. Use of ECG calipers helps demonstrate the regularity of these flutter-waves.

153. **Ventricular escape rhythm ("idioventricular rhythm"), rate 37, peaked T-waves consistent with hyperkalemia.** This patient's serum potassium level was 10·2 mEq/L (normal 3·5–5·3 mEq/L). Hyperkalemia is associated with many ECG changes, including peaked T-waves, PR-interval prolongation and eventual loss of the P-wave (even in the presence of continued sinus node activity), widening of the QRS complex, fascicular and bundle branch blocks, prolonged ventricular pauses on the ECG, and ventricular tachydysrhythmias. It is important to note that the relationship between serum potassium levels and ECG changes may vary significantly between different patients.

154. **ST, rate 170.** The main diagnostic considerations in this narrow-complex regular tachycardia are ST, SVT, and atrial flutter. Although the rhythm might easily be misinterpreted as SVT, the clue that this is ST lies in the T-wave morphology in leads V3–V5: the irregular appearance, or "camel hump," indicates that a P-wave is buried within. There is no evidence of flutter-waves in any of the leads. This patient had ST due to severe hemorrhage from a ruptured ectopic pregnancy.

155. **SR, rate 62, acute lateral MI versus ventricular aneurysm.** The presence of Q-waves with persistent ST-segment elevation indicates MI with ongoing ischemia. An unusual characteristic of this apparent acute MI, however, is the absence of reciprocal ST-segment depression in any of the leads. Although the absence of reciprocal changes certainly does not exclude the diagnosis of acute MI, it at least warrants consideration of an alternative diagnosis (for example ventricular aneurysm, acute pericarditis, BER, etc.) in any patient with ST-segment elevations; and it should prompt efforts to locate previous ECGs for comparison. In this case, the presence of large Q-waves in the lateral leads and the concave-upward morphology of the ST-segments make ventricular aneurysm the only plausible alternative diagnosis besides acute MI. A previous ECG was located and showed similar Q-waves and ST-segments. An echocardiogram confirmed the presence of a ventricular aneurysm and her workup showed no evidence of acute cardiac ischemia.

156. **SR, rate 81, low voltage, LPFB, non-specific T-wave flattening in limb leads.** The most notable finding on this ECG is the presence of low voltage, which was new in comparison to a previous ECG. Low voltage is generally defined as QRS amplitudes <5 mm in all of the limb leads or QRS amplitudes <10 mm in all of the precordial leads. The differential diagnosis for low voltage includes myxedema, large pericardial effusion, large pleural effusion, end-stage cardiomyopathy, severe chronic obstructive pulmonary disease, severe obesity, infiltrative myocardial diseases, constrictive pericarditis, and prior massive MI. In this case, the patient's low voltage was caused by a very large left-sided pleural effusion due to lung cancer. The QRS amplitudes increased after a thoracentesis.

157. **SR with AV dissociation, accelerated AV junctional rhythm, rate 90, capture beats, non-specific T-wave flattening in inferior leads.** Atrial activity and ventricular activity occur independently and the PR-intervals are variable, i.e. AV dissociation is present. Sinus activity occurs at a rate of 75/minute. The atrial complexes are difficult to identify at times in this ECG because they are similar in size to the T-waves. However, use of ECG calipers makes identification of the atrial rhythm easier. Note that some of the P-waves are "buried" within the T-waves, causing those T-waves to have a "pointed" appearance at the top. The QRS complexes are narrow, indicating an AV junctional origin. Because the ventricular rate is faster than the intrinsic rate of the AV junction (normally 40–60/minute), the rhythm is referred to as an "accelerated" AV junctional rhythm. Note that the QRS complexes occur **irregularly** because the eighth and 14th complexes occur early. This early activation of the ventricle is likely the result of sinus P-waves that are conducted. These

are referred to as "capture" beats and indicates that third degree (complete) heart block is **not** present. Recall that when complete heart block is present, **none** of the P-waves get conducted (there should be no capture beats) and the QRS complexes occur **regularly**.

158. **SR, rate 60, high left ventricular voltage, abnormal Q-waves in lateral leads suggestive of hypertrophic cardiomyopathy (HCM).** HCM is often associated with characteristic ECG findings, including large-amplitude QRS complexes, deep narrow Q-waves in the inferior and/or lateral leads mimicking inferior and/or lateral MI, and tall R-waves in leads V1 – V2 that mimic PMI or RVH. The ECG abnormalities are presumed to be caused by ventricular septal hypertrophy. The deep narrow Q-waves are perhaps the most specific of the abnormalities, often leading to the misdiagnosis of MI. However, the Q-waves associated with MI tend to be wider (≥0·04 seconds). The term "high left ventricular voltage" (HLVV) is often used in patients under the age of 40 with large-amplitude QRS complexes. "LVH" implies the existence of an abnormal condition; on the contrary, many normal healthy adolescents and young adults manifest large-amplitude QRS complexes on ECG.

159. **Atrial flutter with 2:1 AV conduction, rate 150, LVH.** The rhythm is narrow-complex and regular; the main considerations are ST, SVT, and atrial flutter. Whenever the ventricular rate is 150 ± 20, atrial flutter should always be strongly considered and all 12 leads should be scrutinized for the presence of flutter-waves. In this case, as in many others, the traditional lead II rhythm strip does not provide an obvious answer. However, leads III and aVF display evidence of atrial activity at a rate of 150/minute and 2:1 AV conduction. LVH can be diagnosed when the amplitude of the R-wave in lead V5 or V6 >26 mm.

160. **ST with AV dissociation and third degree AV block, AV junctional rhythm with incomplete RBBB, rate 40, ST-segment depressions consistent with anterior ischemia.** There is evidence of AV dissociation–independent atrial (atrial rate 110/minute) and ventricular (ventricular rate 40/minute) activity and constantly varying PR-intervals. There is no evidence that any of the P-waves are conducted to the ventricle, thus third degree AV block is diagnosed. The QRS-interval is <0·12 seconds; therefore, a ventricular escape rhythm is unlikely. Rather, an AV junctional rhythm is diagnosed. The QRS complexes have an RBBB morphology but because the QRS-interval is <0·12 seconds, incomplete RBBB is diagnosed.

161. **SR with frequent PACs, rate 89, low voltage.** This rhythm was initially misdiagnosed as second degree AV block because of the intermittent pauses in the rhythm. In order for second degree AV block to be diagnosed, the P-P interval should be constant. In this case, however, the fourth, sixth and 13th QRS complexes are preceded by P-waves that occur **early** in the cycle. Each of the PACs is followed by a pause. Low voltage is diagnosed based on the presence of QRS amplitudes <10 mm in all of the precordial leads and was attributable to obesity.

162. **Probable ST, rate 121, LBBB.** The differential diagnosis for a wide-complex regular rhythm includes VT, ST with aberrant conduction, SVT with aberrant conduction, and atrial flutter with aberrant conduction. Close inspection of all 12 leads reveals the presence of subtle P-waves in lead V1 that have a 1:1 relationship with the QRS complexes; therefore, an atrial tachycardia is diagnosed. In order to be certain that this is **sinus** tachycardia (as opposed to an ectopic atrial tachycardia), upright P-waves would have to be identified in lead I and in the inferior leads.

163. **ST, rate 159, rightward axis and prolonged QT suggestive of cyclic antidepressant overdose.** Cyclic antidepressant overdoses cause characteristic ECG changes that should be recognized by all emergency physicians: tachycardia, rightward axis, tall R-wave in lead aVR, prolonged QT and/or QTc, and widening of the QRS-interval. This ECG demonstrates all of these findings except QRS-interval widening. Treatment with intravenous sodium bicarbonate resulted in resolution of all ECG abnormalities. The patient in this case later admitted to overdose of amitriptyline.

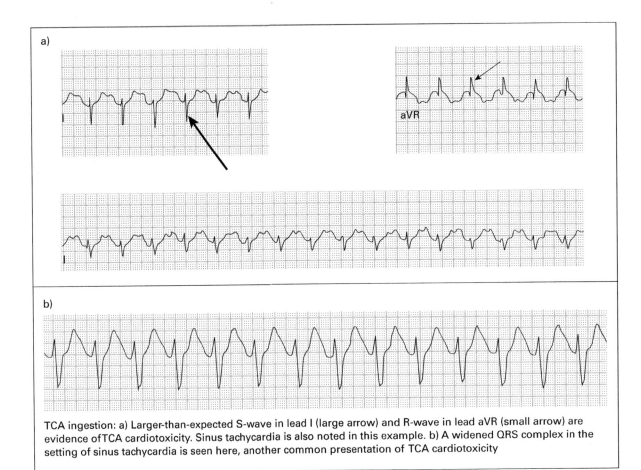

TCA ingestion: a) Larger-than-expected S-wave in lead I (large arrow) and R-wave in lead aVR (small arrow) are evidence of TCA cardiotoxicity. Sinus tachycardia is also noted in this example. b) A widened QRS complex in the setting of sinus tachycardia is seen here, another common presentation of TCA cardiotoxicity

164. **ST, rate 134, inferior MI of uncertain age, T-wave abnormality consistent with inferior and anterior ischemia.** Q-wave in the inferior leads in association with T-wave inversions in the same leads is suggestive of a recent MI or a previous MI with new ischemia. Review of a previous ECG demonstrated that the Q-waves were old but the T-wave inversions were new. As discussed earlier, simultaneous T-wave inversions in the inferior and anteroseptal leads should prompt consideration of pulmonary embolism. In this case, the patient was treated for acute cardiac ischemia without resolution of the T-wave abnormality. He had an emergency coronary angiogram that showed no evidence of acute coronary obstruction. Finally, pulmonary embolism was considered; he then underwent computerized tomography of the lungs that demonstrated several large pulmonary emboli.

165. **SR, rate 67, high left ventricular voltage, prolonged QT and T-wave abnormality suggestive of electrolyte abnormality.** The QT-interval is 0·548 seconds and the QTc is 0·579 seconds. The T-waves have a "camel hump" appearance in some leads. The combination of an apparent prolonged QT-interval and the abnormal T-wave morphology is the result of fusion of the T-wave with the U-wave, a finding typical of hypokalemia. This patient's serum potassium level was 3·0 mEq/L (normal 3·5–5·3 mEq/L).

166. **Atrial fibrillation with AV dissociation and third degree AV block, AV junctional escape rhythm, rate 49, digoxin effect, probable digoxin toxicity.** The ECG has many characteristics that, when taken together, are pathognomonic of digoxin toxicity. The underlying atrial rhythm is atrial fibrillation, evident in several leads that show fine, low amplitude fibrillatory waves. The patient's prior history of chronic atrial fibrillation also supports this. Atrial fibrillation is normally associated with an irregularly irregular ventricular response because

of the random conduction of atrial impulses to the ventricle. The ventricular response in this case, however, is **regular**, a finding that could only be present if the fibrillatory waves are completely blocked from reaching the ventricle (third degree AV heart block, due to digoxin toxicity) and instead an AV junctional or ventricular focus has become the new pacemaker. The rhythm is narrow-complex (the QRS-interval is difficult to measure because of the slurred downstroke of the R-wave leading into the T-wave; the best leads, in this case, to measure the QRS-interval are leads V4 or V5). The narrow QRS complexes and the rate (49/minute) suggests an AV junctional rhythm. The slurred downstroke of the R-waves leading into the T-waves gives a "hockey-stick" appearance (some people refer to this as having the appearance of Salvadore Dali's moustache). This appearance is often associated with digoxin use and is referred to as "digoxin effect." In general digoxin toxicity should be strongly suspected whenever atrial fibrillation is associated with a slow regular ventricle response. This patient's serum digoxin level was 5·1 ng/ml (normal 0·5–2·2 ng/ml).

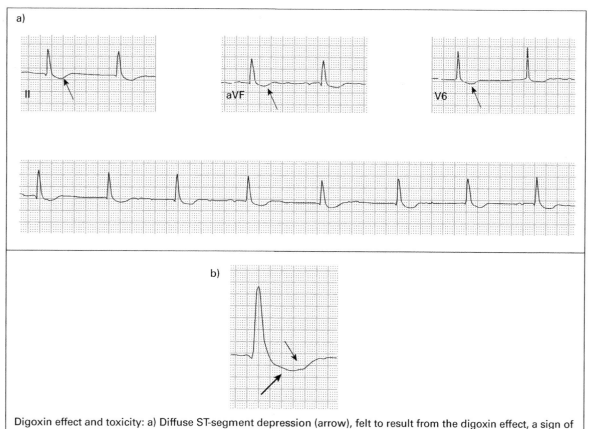

Digoxin effect and toxicity: a) Diffuse ST-segment depression (arrow), felt to result from the digoxin effect, a sign of "adequate digitilization of the heart," not indicative of toxicity. The only evidence of digoxin toxicity seen here is the bradyarrhythmia (junctional rhythm) with atrioventricular dissociation (seen on the 12-lead ECG). b) ST-segment depression, felt to result from the digoxin effect – a nontoxic ECG manifestation. The morphology of the ST-segment depression is highly characteristic of the digoxin effect. In this example, the ST-segment is depressed in a downsloping manner (large arrow) with a gradually increasing depression and more rapid return of the depressed segment to the baseline (small arrow)

167.   **ST, rate 123, low voltage, electrical alternans, findings diagnostic of large pericardial effusion.** The ECG demonstrates findings that are diagnostic of a large pericardial effusion: tachycardia, low voltage, and electrical alternans. Low voltage is associated with large pericardial effusions, myxedema, large pleural effusions, end-stage cardiomyopathy, severe chronic obstructive pulmonary disease, severe obesity, infiltrative myocardial diseases, constrictive pericarditis, and prior massive MI. **New** low voltage, especially in the presence of tachycardia, should strongly suggest the presence of a large pericardial effusion. Electrical alternans, variations in the amplitudes of the QRS complexes, is not specific for pericardial effusion. However,

its presence in the setting of low voltage is highly specific for large pericardial effusions. Electrical alternans is presumed to be caused by the pendular motion of the heart within the fluid-filled pericardial sac. This patient had developed a large pericardial effusion with pericardial tamponade.

168. **SR with frequent premature junctional complexes (PJCs) in a pattern of junctional trigeminy, rate 79, prolonged QT.** The rhythm strip demonstrates "grouped beating": the QRS complexes appear in groups of three, separated by short pauses. Grouped beating should always prompt consideration of second degree AV block versus premature complexes. Second degree AV block is characterized by regular P-P intervals whereas premature beats occur early. In this ECG, inverted P-waves precede the early QRS complexes. The PR-interval in these P-QRS complexes is <0·12 seconds, which suggests that these premature beats arise from the AV junction (PJCs) rather than from the atria (PACs). The prolonged QT-interval was attributed to mild hypomagnesemia. The QT-interval prolongation and the PJCs resolved after supplemental magnesium was administered.

169. **SR with AV dissociation, AV junctional rhythm, occasional capture beats, rate 42, T-wave abnormality consistent with inferior ischemia.** The underlying atrial rhythm is SR with sinus arrhythmia; the atrial rate is 68/minute. The P-P intervals are mostly constant, the PR-intervals are variable, there is evidence of non-conducted P-waves; these all indicate that AV dissociation is present. The first, third, fourth, sixth and seventh QRS complexes represent an AV junctional rhythm; the complexes are narrow and have a rate of 40/minute. The underlying rhythm, however, is interrupted by two narrow QRS complexes (the second and fifth beats), occurring early and each preceded by a P-wave. These QRS complexes are likely the result of ventricular activation by the preceding P-waves, or "capture beats." Because these atrial impulses are being conducted, this is **not** considered third degree (complete) heart block, i.e. this is an example of AV dissociation **without** third degree heart block. These conducted beats cause the sinus node to "reset," causing the next P-wave to occur early. Whenever AV dissociation is present and the escape rhythm is interrupted by an early, narrow QRS complex, consider the possibility that these are capture beats (therefore third degree heart block is absent).

170. **Accelerated ventricular rhythm, rate 90.** Normal sinus P-waves are absent in this rhythm. In fact, retrograde P-waves are noted in several leads. The absence of sinus P-waves and the rightward axis in this wide-complex rhythm supports the diagnosis of a ventricular rhythm. A ventricular rhythm that has a rate between 40/minute and 110–115/minute is referred to as an "accelerated" ventricular rhythm, or "accelerated idioventricular rhythm" (AIVR). AIVR is a common rhythm that occurs in patients that receive thrombolytics after an acute MI. The rhythm is presumed to be a marker of reperfusion. The AIVR usually is self-terminating within minutes. Treatment with antidysrhythmics may induce asystole.

171. **Atrial fibrillation with slow ventricular response versus AV junctional bradycardia, rate 20, peaked T-waves consistent with hyperkalemia.** Prominent T-waves are noted in many leads. Prominent T-waves may be found in acute myocardial ischemia, hyperkalemia, acute pericarditis, LVH, BER, bundle branch block, and pre-excitation syndromes. The T-waves of hyperkalemia are usually narrow-based, as seen in this example, whereas in the other conditions noted above they usually have a broader base. Hyperkalemia can be associated with bradydysrhythmias, including slow sinus, AV junctional, and ventricular rhythms. Prolonged pauses can also occur, as seen here. Hyperkalemia does not usually cause atrial fibrillation, however, thus casting some doubt on the diagnosis of atrial fibrillation in this irregular rhythm. The patient in this case had developed new renal failure from severe dehydration and sepsis. Her serum potassium level was 7·4 mEq/L (normal 3·5–5·3 mEq/L). She was treated with intravenous calcium, sodium bicarbonate, and insulin with prompt return to sinus rhythm. Hyperkalemia should always be considered in patients with extreme bradycardia and absent P-waves.

172. **ST, rate 124, acute inferior and right ventricular (RV) MI.** Q-waves and ST-segment elevation in the inferior leads indicates acute MI. RV extension of the MI is diagnosed based on the presence of simultaneous ST-segment elevation in lead V1 and ST-segment depression in lead V2. RV MI was confirmed using right-sided chest leads and echocardiography. Reciprocal ST-segment depression is noted in the lateral leads.

173. **Atrial flutter with 2:1 AV conduction, rate 130.** Although the classic "sawtooth" pattern is absent, atrial flutter is diagnosed based on the presence of atrial complexes at a rate of 260/minute in the inferior leads. Interestingly, the ECG computer misinterpreted the rhythm as ST with acute inferior MI because of what appears to be ST-segment elevation in the inferior leads. The apparent ST-segment elevation is simply the result of atrial complexes that are fused to the terminal portion of the QRS complex.

174. **SR, rate 66, T-wave abnormality in aVL suggestive of acute inferior ischemia or early infarction.** Lead aVL is perhaps the most common lead in which reciprocal abnormalities occur in the setting of acute inferior myocardial ischemia and infarction. The reciprocal abnormalities can consist of T-wave inversions and/or ST-segment depression. These abnormalities can actually precede the development of ischemic findings in the inferior leads.[5] Isolated T-wave inversions and/or ST-segment depression in lead aVL, therefore, should not be ignored; it would be prudent to observe these patients and obtain serial ECGs to monitor for ST-segment and T-wave abnormalities in the inferior leads.

175. **SB, rate 55, acute inferior MI with possible right ventricular (RV) extension.** This ECG was obtained from the same patient as in case #174 approximately two hours later. Acute MI is indicated by the presence of ST-segment elevation. Reciprocal ST-segment depression and T-wave inversions are noted in leads I and aVL, typical of acute inferior MI. One will note more marked abnormalities that are now found in lead aVL compared to those found in ECG #174. RV extension of the MI is suggested by the presence of ST-segment elevation in lead III that is more pronounced than the ST-segment elevation found in lead II.

176. **ST, rate 114, acute pericarditis with probable large pericardial effusion.** The ECG was initially misdiagnosed as acute inferior MI. However, there are several clues that suggest the alternative diagnosis.
    - ST-segment elevation in the inferior leads is associated with mild PR-segment depression, a finding highly specific for acute pericarditis.
    - Slight PR-segment elevation is present in lead aVR, suggestive of (though not specific to) acute pericarditis.
    - The QRS voltage is low (although the **formal** criteria for diagnosis is not met).
    - Electrical alternans is present in some areas of the ECG, including lead V1.
    - Reciprocal ST-segment depression, common with acute MI, is absent.

    Intravenous anticoagulants were administered to this patient for presumed cardiac ischemia; pericardial tamponade resulted. The patient required immediate reversal of anticoagulation and emergent pericardiotomy, after which he did well.

177. **Marked SB with frequent PVCs in a pattern of ventricular bigeminy, rate 56.** Acute ischemic or hemorrhagic strokes are associated with many ECG abnormalities, including ventricular ectopy, tachy- or bradydysrhythmias, AV blocks, ST-segment elevation or depression, prolonged QT-interval, and large inverted T-waves. Various theories have been proposed for these abnormalities although no single cause has been found. CNS events that produce elevated intracranial pressure are especially likely to produce these abnormalities.

178. **SR with intermittent runs of non-sustained VT, VT rate 150.** The first QRS complex is narrow and preceded by upright P-waves in lead I, II, and III indicating underlying sinus rhythm. The rhythm then becomes VT (P-waves are found within some of the T-waves, indicating AV dissociation); after an 8-beat run of VT, sinus rhythm recurs for two beats, then another run of VT begins. VT is defined as a ventricular rhythm of ≥3 beats at a rate >110–120/minute. If the rhythm lasts ≤30 seconds, it generally is referred to as non-sustained VT; if >30 seconds, it is referred to as sustained VT.

179. **ST with frequent premature junctional complexes (PJCs) in a pattern of junctional trigeminy, rate 110, PRWP.** Grouped beating in triplets is present. Grouped beats should always prompt consideration of second degree AV block versus premature complexes. The third QRS complex in every triplet is preceded by a

P-wave that occurs early and with a different morphology, ruling out second degree AV block in favor of premature complexes. The premature complexes likely arise from the AV junction rather than an ectopic atrial focus because the PR-interval is <0·12 seconds. This patient's laboratory workup was notable for mild hypokalemia and hypomagnesemia. With potassium and magnesium supplementation, the premature complexes resolved.

180. **MAT, rate 115, RBBB.** The main considerations with any wide-complex, irregular tachycardia include atrial fibrillation with aberrant conduction (for example bundle branch block), atrial flutter with variable block and aberrant conduction, MAT with aberrant conduction, atrial fibrillation with WPW, and polymorphic ventricular tachycardia. P-waves are noted in the rhythm strip; they occur irregularly, are followed by QRS complexes without evidence of non-conducted beats, and are of various morphologies. These findings are typical of MAT. A RBBB is present, accounting for the wide QRS complexes.

181. **Possible atrial fibrillation, rate 90, non-specific intraventricular conduction delay.** The rhythm is irregular with QRS complexes of a markedly wide, bizarre morphology. Extremely rapid wide-complex tachycardias with bizarre-shaped QRS morphologies should suggest atrial fibrillation with WPW. When the rhythm is slower, however, hyperkalemia should be strongly considered. Hyperkalemia can cause various ECG abnormalities, including ventricular tachydysrhythmias and bradydysrhythmias. The markedly wide and unusually-shaped QRS complexes are typical of severe hyperkalemia and indicate a pre-sine wave or pre-arrest state. This patient had developed new renal failure, presumably caused by diabetes and recent prolonged use of non-steroidal anti-inflammatory medications. Her serum potassium was 8·3 mEq/L (normal 3·5–5·3 mEq/L). A rightward axis is often associated with severe hyperkalemia and normalizes with treatment.

182. **SR, rate 70, incomplete RBBB with ST-segment elevation in right precordial leads consistent with the Brugada syndrome.** As discussed in cases #111 and #131, the Brugada syndrome is characterized by an incomplete or complete RBBB pattern with ST-segment elevation in the right precordial leads. The condition is associated with a predisposition to development of VT, especially polymorphic VT. Patients with a presumptive diagnosis of the Brugada syndrome based on ECG should be referred for electrophysiology studies for definitive diagnosis and, if positive, placement of an internal cardioverter-defibrillator. This patient's ECG diagnosis was made in retrospect – soon after her discharge from the emergency department she collapsed. Medics were called and found her pulseless with PVT. Resuscitation efforts were unsuccessful.

183. **SB, rate 46, LVH, J-waves suggestive of hypothermia.** This patient had sepsis with acute adrenal insufficiency, hypoglycemia, and hypothermia. His rectal temperature was 30·9 degrees Celsius (87·6 degrees Fahrenheit). J- ("Osborne") waves are noted in the lateral precordial leads and produce the appearance of ST-segment elevation. SB is common in mild to moderate hypothermia.

184. **SB with frequent PVCs in a pattern of ventricular bigeminy, rate 90, T-wave abnormality consistent with inferior and anterior ischemia.** The sinus rate is 45/minute. Ventricular bigeminy is present. Close attention to the T-waves that are associated with the normal QRS complexes reveals T-wave inversions in the inferior and anterior leads. These T-wave inversions resolved after the patient was treated with nitroglycerin. A stress test performed later demonstrated cardiac ischemia.

185. **SR with AV dissociation, AV junctional rhythm, rate 35, occasional capture beats, bifascicular block (RBBB and LAFB), LVH, T-wave abnormality consistent with inferior ischemia.** The sinus rate is 97/minute but the ventricular rate is 35/minute. The PR-intervals vary, consistent with AV dissociation. The QRS complexes occur regularly except for the very last QRS complex, which occurs early, has a different morphology, and is preceded by a P-wave with a normal PR-interval. These are indications that the final QRS complex is a capture beat. The presence of a capture beat indicates that third degree (complete) heart block is **not** present.

186. **Ectopic atrial rhythm, rate 69, high left ventricular voltage, abnormal Q-waves in lateral leads suggestive of hypertrophic cardiomyopathy (HCM).** The inverted P-wave in lead III suggests a non-sinus node origin. The PR-interval is >0·12 seconds, indicating that the P-waves originate from an ectopic atrial focus rather than an AV junctional focus. The large-amplitude QRS complexes are typical of HCM, as are the deep narrow Q-waves in the lateral leads. In this case, the abnormal Q-waves are most notable in leads I and aVL. HCM Q-waves tend to be narrower than MI Q-waves, which usually are ≥0·04 seconds wide. This patient had been evaluated on two other occasions for exertional syncope. During both of those physician visits, ECGs were obtained and demonstrated similar findings. However, the ECG abnormalities went unrecognized until his current visit.

187. **SR with second degree AV block and 2:1 AV conduction, rate 46, acute inferior MI.** Regular P-waves at a rate of 92/minute are found easily in the inferior leads. There is a 2:1 ratio of P-waves:QRS complexes, and the PR-interval remains constant, consistent with second degree AV block. When second degree AV block occurs with 2:1 AV conduction, the diagnosis of Mobitz I versus Mobitz II cannot be certain, although the narrow QRS complexes favors Mobitz I. Q-waves with ST-segment elevation is present in the inferior leads. Reciprocal ST-segment depression is found in I, aVL, and V2–4.

188. **SB with frequent non-conducted PACs in a pattern of atrial bigeminy, rate 45, bifascicular block (RBBB and LAFB).** The rhythm was initially misdiagnosed as second degree AV block with 2:1 AV conduction because there are two P-waves for every QRS complex, similar to the previous example (#187). Unlike the previous example, however, the P-waves do **not** occur regularly. Therefore, second degree AV block is essentially ruled out. The first P-wave in each cycle is a sinus P-wave. This is followed by a QRS complex, then a non-conducted P-wave (a non-conducted PAC). One will note that the PACs have a slightly different morphology to the sinus P-waves. PACs that occur too early in the cycle (before the ventricle has "reset") do not produce ventricular depolarization. Instead, they are followed by a pause before the next atrial beat occurs. This can easily lead to a misdiagnosis of second degree AV block.

189. **SR, rate 75, T-wave abnormality consistent with anteroseptal ischemia.** Although cardiac ischemia is a common cause of T-wave inversions, other conditions are associated with this abnormality as well: persistent juvenile T-wave patterns, left ventricular hypertrophy, acute myocarditis, WPW syndrome, cerebrovascular accident, bundle branch block, later stages of pericarditis, and acute pulmonary embolism. T-wave inversions in the right precordial leads are especially common in pulmonary embolism, with sensitivities for this finding as high as 50%. In this case, the physician initiated treatment for acute cardiac ischemia. However, neither the T-wave inversions nor the chest pain resolved with the administration of nitroglycerin or heparin. At that point, computerized tomography of the lungs with intravenous contrast was performed and demonstrated three pulmonary emboli. Acute pulmonary embolism should always be considered when the ECG demonstrates new T-wave inversions, especially when they are present in the right precordial leads.

190. **Atrial tachycardia with variable AV block, rate 72, lateral MI of uncertain age, non-specific intraventricular conduction delay, rhythm suggestive of digoxin toxicity.** The atrial rate, best noted in lead V1, is 200/minute. Atrial tachycardia with variable AV block ("PAT with block") is highly specific for digoxin toxicity. The serum digoxin level in this case was 4·7 ng/ml (normal 0·5–2·2 ng/ml).

191. **SR, rate 82, RAE, non-specific T-wave flattening in inferior leads, abnormal precordial T-wave balance.** The normal ECG has an inverted, flat, or small upright T-wave in lead V1. The T-wave usually is upright in lead V2 and becomes larger in the other precordial leads in normal ECGs. In this case, however, the T-wave in lead V1 is not only upright, but it is larger than the T-waves in the lateral leads. Marriott has referred to this abnormality as "abnormal T-wave balance."[5] Marriott and other others[6,7] have suggested that when the T-wave in lead V1 is upright and large (more specifically, when the T-wave in lead V1 is larger than the T-wave in lead V6), it suggests underlying cardiac disease. This patient did prove to have a 90% obstructing lesion of the LAD.

149

192. **SR, rate 64, RAE, non-specific T-wave flattening in the inferior leads, T-wave abnormality in the anterior leads consistent with acute anterior ischemia.** This ECG was obtained on the same patient as in case #191 when symptoms recurred 12 hours later. The ECG demonstrates Wellens' sign – biphasic T-waves in the mid-precordial leads. Wellens' sign is a highly specific marker of proximal LAD disease. The T-wave abnormality often occurs even in the absence of chest pain. This patient had emergent coronary angiography, which demonstrated a 90% obstructing proximal LAD lesion. The T-wave abnormality resolved after angioplasty.

193. **SR, rate 74, inferior MI of uncertain age, acute anterior MI versus ventricular aneurysm, low voltage.** The presence of Q-waves with persistent ST-segment elevation in the anterior leads is most likely due to MI with ongoing ischemia. However, the absence of reciprocal ST-depression in other leads should prompt consideration of ventricular aneurysm as an alternative diagnosis. Efforts should be made to obtain previous ECGs for comparison to determine if the Q-waves and ST-segment elevation are new or old. In this case, a previous ECG was obtained and showed similar abnormalities. An emergent echocardiogram was obtained and demonstrated evidence of a large left ventricular aneurysm. Low voltage is due to the prior massive MI.

194. **AV junctional rhythm with occasional premature junctional complexes (PJCs) in a pattern of junctional trigeminy, rate 40, peaked T-waves suggestive of hyperkalemia.** Careful evaluation of the ECG reveals that the rhythm is regularly irregular. The QRS complexes are narrow and occur in groups of three. The first two QRS complexes of each group occur at a rate of 46/minute and have no preceding P-waves, suggesting an AV junctional rhythm. The third QRS complex of each group occurs early and has no preceding P-wave, indicating that it is a PJC. The groups of beats are separated by markedly prolonged pauses. The prolonged pauses, the absence of P-waves, and the peaking of the T-waves are all suggestive of hyperkalemia. This patient's serum potassium level was 7·9 mEq/L (normal 3·5–5·3 mEq/L).

195. **ST, rate 105, low voltage.** Low voltage is defined by QRS amplitudes in all of the limb leads <5 mm or in all of the precordial leads <10 mm. The differential diagnosis of low voltage includes myxedema, large pericardial effusion, large pleural effusion, end-stage cardiomyopathy, severe chronic obstructive pulmonary disease, severe obesity, infiltrative myocardial diseases, constrictive pericarditis, and prior massive MI. The combination of low voltage plus tachycardia should prompt early consideration of a large pericardial effusion. The patient in this case had an urgent echocardiogram, which demonstrated a large pericardial effusion and tamponade. Bacteria were cultured from the pericardial fluid and blood. Despite pericardiotomy and treatment with intravenous antibiotics, he died of sepsis.

196. **SR, rate 85, LBBB, ST-segment abnormality consistent with acute ischemia or MI.** ST-segment depression in lead V3 meets the Sgarbossa[8] criteria for acute MI (see case #95). The magnitude of ST-segment depression in the lateral precordial leads is unusual in LBBB and is also suggestive of acute ischemia. This patient ruled out for acute MI but did prove to have acute ischemia based on stress testing.

197. **AV junctional rhythm, rate 50, LVH, non-specific T-wave flattening diffusely.** There is no evidence of sinus node or other atrial activity, therefore an atrial rhythm is excluded. The QRS complexes are narrow, suggesting an AV junctional rhythm rather than a ventricular rhythm. The rate of 50/minute is also typical of an AV junctional rhythm. This patient was already regularly taking a calcium channel blocking medication when she was prescribed a beta-receptor blocking medication. Her lightheadedness started the day after she began taking the second medication.

198. **Atrial flutter with variable block, rate 80, reversal of V1 and V2 electrodes.** The rhythm was initially misdiagnosed as atrial fibrillation because of the irregularly irregular rhythm. The rhythm strip does not demonstrate obvious regular atrial activity. However, lead III does demonstrate a classic flutter-wave appearance. Abnormal precordial T-wave balance (i.e. lead V1 has an abnormally large T-wave in comparison to the other precordial leads) and abnormal R-wave progression (i.e. the R-waves in leads V1–V3 do not

gradually enlarge) are noted. Both of these abnormalities are accounted for because of reversal of the V1 and V2 electrodes. Flutter-waves are noted in the correct lead V1.

199. **SR with frequent PACs in a pattern of atrial bigeminy and occasional PVCs, rate 88.** Groups (pairs) of beats are present. As discussed previously, grouped-beating should always prompt consideration of second degree AV block versus premature beats. Second degree AV block will be associated with regular atrial activity (constant P-P intervals). In this case, however, the P-waves (best noted in lead V1) are irregular. The second beat in each pair is a PAC.

200. **ST, rate 108, prolonged QT, ST-segment and T-wave abnormality consistent with diffuse cardiac ischemia versus intracranial hemorrhage.** The combination of a prolonged QT-interval with deeply inverted wide T-waves should prompt immediate consideration of a large intracranial hemorrhage with elevated intracranial pressure (ICP). Although acute cardiac ischemia can occasionally produce large wide inverted T-waves, the mental status of these patients should be normal. The exact cause of the T-wave abnormality associated with elevated ICP is not definitively known. One theory is that intracranial hemorrhage with elevated ICP causes increased vagal tone, which produces aberrant repolarization. Another theory is that massive catecholamine discharge occurs, leading to severe coronary vasoconstriction and ischemia. Acute cerebrovascular events are also associated with tachydysrhythmias, bradydysrhythmias, AV blocks, and ST-segment changes (elevation or depression). The patient in this case had a large intracranial hemorrhage due to a brain metastasis.

References

1. Brugada P, Brugada J. Right bundle branch block, persistent ST-segment elevation and sudden cardiac death: A distinct clinical and electrocardiographic syndrome. *J Am Coll Cardiol* 1992;**20**:1391–6.
2. Brugada P, Brugada R, Brugada J. The Brugada syndrome. *Curr Cardiol Rep* 2000;**2**:507–14.
3. Yamaji H, Iwasaki K, Kusachi S *et al.* Prediction of acute left main coronary artery obstruction by 12-lead electrocardiography. *J Am Coll Cardiol* 2001;**38**:1348–54.
4. Zema, MJ. Electrocardiographic tall R waves in the right precordial leads. *J Electrocardiol* 1990;**23**:147–56.
5. Marriott HJ. *Emergency Electrocardiography*. Naples, FL: Trinity Press, 1997, pp. 28–36.
6. Barthwal SP, Agarwal R, Sarkari NB *et al.* Diagnostic significance of T I < T III and TV1 > TV6 signs in ischaemic heart disease. *J Assoc Phys India* 1993;**41**:26–7.
7. Manno BV, Hakki AH, Iskandrian AS, Hare T. Significance of the upright T wave in precordial lead V1 in adults with coronary artery disease. *J Am Coll Cardiol* 1983;**1**:1213–15.
8. Sgarbossa EB, Pinski SL, Barbagelata A *et al.* Electrocardiographic diagnosis of evolving acute myocardial infarction in the presence of left bundle-branch block, GUSTO-1 (Global Utilization of Streptokinase and Tissue Plasminogen Activator for Occluded Coronary Arteries) Investigators. *N Engl J Med* 1996;**334**:481–7.

Appendix A

Differential diagnoses

Diffuse ST-segment elevation
Large AMI, acute pericarditis, benign early repolarization, ventricular aneurysm, coronary vasospasm

Leftward axis
LAFB, LBBB, inferior myocardial infarction, left ventricular hypertrophy, ventricular ectopy, paced beats, and Wolff-Parkinson-White syndrome

Low voltage
Myxedema, large pericardial effusion, large pleural effusion, end-stage cardiomyopathy, severe chronic obstructive pulmonary disease, severe obesity, infiltrative myocardial diseases, constrictive pericarditis, and prior massive MI

Increased QRS-interval
Hypothermia, hyperkalemia, WPW, aberrant intraventricular conduction (for example bundle branch block), ventricular ectopy, paced beats, medications (extensive list)

Increased QT-interval (and QTc-interval)
Hypokalemia*, hypomagnesemia, hypocalcemia, acute myocardial ischemia, elevated intracranial pressure, drugs with sodium channel blocking effects (for example cyclic antidepressants, quinidine, etc.), hypothermia, and congenital prolonged QT syndrome

*Hypokalemia is included in this differential diagnosis for consideration; however, the actual QT-interval is normal; the QT-interval **appears** prolonged because of the presence of fusion of the T-wave with a U-wave (a "T-U fusion complex")

Poor R-wave progression (PRWP)
Prior anteroseptal MI, LVH, abnormally high placement of the mid-precordial electrodes, or may simply be a normal variant

Prominent R-wave in lead V_1
WPW, PMI, RBBB (or incomplete RBBB), ventricular ectopy, RVH, acute right ventricular dilatation (right ventricular "strain," for example massive pulmonary embolism), hypertrophic cardiomyopathy, progressive muscular dystrophy, dextrocardia, and misplaced precordial electrodes. The prominent R-wave in lead V_1 (defined as an R:S ratio ≥ 1) exists as a normal variant in only rare instances.

Prominent T-wave
Acute myocardial ischemia, hyperkalemia, acute pericarditis, LVH, BER, bundle branch block, and pre-excitation syndromes

Rightward axis
LPFB, lateral myocardial infarction, right ventricular hypertrophy, acute (for example pulmonary embolism) and chronic (for example emphysema) lung disease, ventricular ectopy, hyperkalemia, overdoses of sodium-channel blocking drugs (for example cyclic antidepressants). Normal young or slender adults with a horizontally positioned heart can also demonstrate a rightward QRS axis on the ECG.

ST-segment elevation in lead V_1
LVH, LBBB, acute anteroseptal MI, acute right ventricular MI, Brugada syndrome, pulmonary embolism

Tachydysrhythmias

Narrow-complex regular rhythm: ST, SVT, atrial flutter

Narrow-complex irregular rhythm: atrial fibrillation, atrial flutter with variable block, MAT

Wide-complex regular rhythm: VT, ST with aberrant conduction, SVT with aberrant conduction, atrial flutter with aberrant conduction

Wide-complex irregular rhythm: atrial fibrillation with aberrant conduction (for example bundle branch block), atrial flutter with variable block and aberrant conduction, MAT with aberrant conduction, atrial fibrillation with WPW, polymorphic ventricular tachycardia

Appendix B

Commonly used abbreviations

AIVR	accelerated idioventricular rhythm
AMI	acute myocardial infarction
BER	benign early repolarization
HCM	hypertrophic cardiomyopathy
LAD	left anterior descending artery
LAE	left atrial enlargement
LAFB	left anterior fascicular block
LBBB	left bundle branch block
LPFB	left posterior fascicular block
LVH	left ventricular hypertrophy
MAT	multifocal atrial activity
MI	myocardial infarction
PAC	premature atrial contraction
PAT	paroxysmal atrial tachycardia
PMI	posterior myocardial infarction
PRWP	poor R-wave progression
PS	pacemaker "spike"
PVC	premature ventricular contraction
RBBB	right bundle branch block
RVH	right ventricular hypertrophy
SB	sinus bradycardia
SR	sinus rhythm
ST	sinus tachycardia
SVT	supraventricular tachycardia
VT	ventricular tachycardia
WPW	Wolff-Parkinson-White syndrome

Index

Printed and bound by CPI Group (UK) Ltd, Croydon, CR0 4YY

16/05/2024

14503473-0001

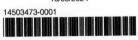